NATURAL
SOLUTIONS
TO
PCOS

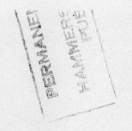

To Verity, the charity for PCOS, for all the good work
you do in supporting women with PCOS

NATURAL
SOLUTIONS
TO
PCOS

HOW TO ELIMINATE YOUR SYMPTOMS AND
BOOST YOUR FERTILITY

MARILYN
GLENVILLE
PhD

MACMILLAN

First published 2012 by Macmillan
an imprint of Pan Macmillan, a division of Macmillan Publishers Limited
Pan Macmillan, 20 New Wharf Road, London N1 9RR
Basingstoke and Oxford
Associated companies throughout the world
www.panmacmillan.com

ISBN 978-0-230-76383-8

1 3 5 7 9 8 6 4 2

A CIP catalogue record for this book is available from the British Library.

Text designed and set by seagulls.net
Printed and bound by CPI Group (UK) Ltd, Croydon, CR0 4YY

This book is intended as a reference volume only, not as a medical manual.
The information given here is designed to help you make informed decisions
about your health. It is not intended as a substitute for any treatment that
you may have been prescribed by your doctor. If you suspect you have
a medical problem, we urge you to seek competent medical help.

Mention of specific companies, organizations or authorities in this book does not
imply endorsement of the publisher, nor does mention of specific companies,
organizations or authorities in the book imply that they endorse the book.

Addresses, websites and telephone numbers given in this book
were correct at the time of going to press.

Visit **www.panmacmillan.com** to read more about all our books
and to buy them. You will also find features, author interviews
and news of any author events, and you can sign up for e-newsletters
so that you're always first to hear about our new releases.

CONTENTS

Acknowledgements   *vii*

Introduction   *1*

PART ONE: PCOS

Chapter 1 What is PCOS?   9

Chapter 2 Diagnosing PCOS   25

Chapter 3 Your Medical Options   31

PART TWO: Natural Solutions to PCOS

Chapter 4 The Seven-Step Diet to Beat PCOS   39

Chapter 5 How to Use Supplements and Herbs   67

Chapter 6 Controlling Your Weight   85

Chapter 7 Exercise   105

Chapter 8 Your Hair and Skin   115

Chapter 9 Stress and PCOS   129

Chapter 10 Environmental Hormone Disruptors   147

PART THREE: Living with PCOS

Chapter 11 Your Fertility   157

Chapter 12 Pregnancy   183

Chapter 13 Nutritional Tests that are Useful in Treating PCOS   191

Chapter 14 Safeguarding Your Future Health   199

Chapter 15 Beyond PCOS   207

Appendix I: Criteria for Diagnosing PCOS   209

Appendix II: Food Nutrient Sources   213

Useful Resources   217

Notes   219

Index   241

ACKNOWLEDGEMENTS

This has been such an important book for me to write as PCOS has become a major problem for many women all around the world and has such an impact on them physically and also psychologically. There is much that can be done to help correct and alleviate the symptoms of PCOS and I am pleased to have the opportunity to share this information here with you.

I would like to thank Liz Gough, my editor and also Cindy Chan and Ali Blackburn at Macmillan, who have been especially helpful in getting this book ready for publication. My thanks also go to Clare Hulton for introducing me to Macmillan and making this book possible.

I am grateful to Louise Atkinson, who has helped to make sure that this book is easy to read and prevented me from getting too bogged down in the medical studies and technical terms.

I would especially like to thank my brilliant team of nutritionists, Alison Belcourt, Helen Heap, Sharon Pitt and Lisa Smith, who work in the London and Tunbridge Wells clinics and who take such good care of our patients. Also to the rest of the team in Tunbridge Wells including Wendy, Brenda, Alex, Gayla, Lee, Dave, Shirley, Felicity and Sarah, who work so diligently behind the scenes making the work I do possible. Thanks also go to my two wonderful nutritionists in Ireland, Heather Leeson and Sally Milne, who are doing a superb job of looking after the women over there.

Special thanks go to all my patients, who have been wonderful in seeking out information on PCOS in order to help themselves. They have shared and talked freely about their symptoms and the impact PCOS has had on their fertility.

Last but not least, my love goes to my family: Kriss, my husband, and my three children Matt (and his wife Hannah and their children Katie and Jack), Len and Chantell (and her partner Phil).

INTRODUCTION

For the past thirty years I have been successfully using natural methods to treat women with a variety of conditions from osteoporosis to hormonal issues such as PMS, irregular, painful and heavy periods, menopause and endometriosis. But some of the most startling and satisfying improvements I have seen have been with women whose lives are blighted by polycystic ovary syndrome (PCOS).

By the time women with PCOS walk through my door they are usually desperate. Many will have tried the various drug options suggested by their doctors, the vast majority will have struggled with diets in a bid to lose weight, but a large number are also depressed and at the end of their tether because they think they'll never be free from the truly horrible symptoms of this condition, or because they face the very real fear that they will never be able to have a baby.

PCOS affects women in so many different ways. In some cases I know exactly what's wrong the moment I see them, while others look completely normal, but inside, their chaotic hormones are wreaking havoc on both their bodies and minds. Invariably, they are miserable, and despairing as to whether they will ever be free from the debilitating symptoms of PCOS.

But after a few tests, some sound advice and a few lifestyle changes, most of the women I see are able to start to turn their lives around. Within three months of following my recommendations, most begin to see positive improvements in their symptoms. Many return for subsequent appointments saying the change is 'miraculous': their skin problems improve, their unwelcome facial and body hair thins and dwindles and most of them see the beginnings of a regular menstrual cycle.

Many women come to me having been told that PCOS means they may never get pregnant, but I have found, time and time again, that if erratic hormones can be settled naturally, fertility will fall into place. In my experience, PCOS certainly does *not* mean you cannot have a baby.

WHO AM I?

I am a registered nutritionist and chartered psychologist and a Fellow of The Royal Society of Medicine and have studied and practised nutrition for thirty years, both in the UK and in the USA.

My focus has always been on the *natural* approach to female hormone problems and, in all my years of practice, I have found that with PCOS, like so many conditions affecting women, the gentle, natural approach works remarkably well.

I believe good diet topped up by supplements and herbs works in harmony with the body, and very often achieves the same effect as drugs, but without any of the potentially negative side effects.

Having said that, many women happily use my recommendations *alongside* their drug treatments. Sometimes the improvements they feel allow them to reduce the dosages of their drugs (in consultation with their doctor, of course), or even come off them completely.

But in all circumstances, whether you are taking prescription drugs or not, my recommendations will help. In the case of IVF, for instance, they can even boost the effectiveness of the fertility drugs and really can increase your chances of having a baby.

Julie's story is very typical of the women I see:

CASE STUDY: JULIE'S STORY

During my early twenties my periods became quite erratic. While I was at university I put this down to stress, but when I reached thirty I noticed that I was also developing more hair around my chin and inner thighs. I had some acne on my back, which was very unusual, as I had always had such clear skin, and I found I was putting on weight rapidly, particularly around my middle.

I saw my GP who diagnosed PCOS and recommended I go on the Pill to regulate my periods. I was reluctant, and asked for more investigations, but he refused.

I did a bit of research and came across the Dr Marilyn Glenville Clinic and booked an appointment with her. We discussed my diet, which, without me realizing, had become very low in fresh food and contained far too many starchy refined carbohydrates, coffee and sugar – these were the foods I had impossible-to-resist cravings for!

She advised that I eat fewer starchy carbohydrates, avoiding them altogether after 6pm, switch to eating plenty of fresh vegetables and protein (fish, eggs, beans, quinoa and nuts and seeds), eliminate or at least reduce my coffee intake to one cup per day and to always have it alongside a meal and not on an empty stomach. She also said that I had to eat every three hours to keep my blood sugar stable, as long gaps would result in fluctuations, which are not conducive to hormonal balance.

She recommended a combination of herbs containing agnus castus, black cohosh and milk thistle to help to lower LH levels (see page 11), support my liver and, hopefully, regulate my cycle. Alongside this, she suggested a good multivitamin and mineral, a fish-oil supplement and additional chromium and zinc.

Within eight weeks of following the diet I noticed I had more energy, my skin seemed to be clearing and I even had a period!

After sixteen weeks, my cycle had started to regulate and I'd lost a significant amount of weight. I was delighted! I had lots of lovely comments from friends and family and this really encouraged me to continue. A year down the line, my hormones are getting back into balance and I now have a regular thirty-two-day cycle. I still have some excess hair, but much lighter in colour so I take this as a very positive sign.

HOW THIS BOOK CAN HELP YOU

I have decided to write this book because my recommendations have helped so many women with PCOS that I now feel really strongly it is time to bring the benefits to women who can't come to see me personally.

If you read this book and take on board my suggestions, you will be doing the best you possibly can to understand PCOS and how it affects you, and you will be able to manage it naturally, with natural solutions that will not do anything to affect adversely the delicate balance of your body.

Although you may have been told that PCOS cannot be cured, you really can be free of symptoms, and the sooner you control your PCOS symptoms the better chance you have of protecting yourself against the potentially long-term damage out-of-control PCOS can have on your health.

You *need* to read this book if you have been given a diagnosis of PCOS and you are looking for answers as to what it means, how it affects your body, your fertility and your long-term health and, most crucially, what you can do about it.

You *should* also read this book if you think you might have PCOS, but are finding it difficult to get a diagnosis and want to know what tests you should be asking for and what it will mean if you do have it.

But, most importantly, you *must* read this book if you have PCOS and you are struggling to get pregnant. Trust me. My methods really do work.

Let's face it, you've got nothing to lose by trying my methods; they are all natural, safe and will only boost your general health. Wouldn't it be a wonderful bonus if they banished your PCOS too? Yes, you'll need to be committed, and some of the nutritional tests and supplements you will have to pay for privately, but believe me, it will be so worth it.

I have divided the book into three parts: Part One tells you everything you need to know about PCOS – what it is, how it is diagnosed and how it is conventionally treated; Part Two offers my unique natural programme of treatment – dietary recommendations and supplements and lifestyle changes to support them; and Part Three deals with coping with the condition long term – how to live with PCOS, how to boost fertility and conceive and how to safeguard your future health.

This book will both inform and inspire you. And, above all, it will give you back control over your body, letting you know that you do not have to put up with PCOS for a single day longer.

Wishing you good health.

Marilyn

PART ONE

PCOS

CHAPTER 1

WHAT IS PCOS?

Polycystic ovary syndrome (PCOS) is a hormonal imbalance that affects an estimated 5 to 10 per cent of women of reproductive age across the world, and results in irregular or absent periods, acne, excess body hair and weight gain. It can also cause problems with fertility.

PCOS gets its name because under an ultrasound scan, the ovaries can look like a bunch of grapes, each one covered in what look like multiple cysts. In fact, these aren't cysts at all, but are small, undeveloped follicles.

Doctors have known of the existence of PCOS for over seventy years – it was first spotted in 1935 and named Stein-Leventhal syndrome after the two doctors who identified it – but although it is the single most common hormonal imbalance in women of reproductive age and a major cause of infertility, it is, even today, still frequently misdiagnosed and often missed completely. As a result, many women suffer on in silence, unaware of the many tests and treatments available and the huge difference a few simple diet and lifestyle changes can make.

The first step to controlling PCOS is understanding what it is and how it works. Only then can you start to break down the interlinking elements and set your life back on track.

SYMPTOMS OF PCOS

Not every woman with PCOS will get the same symptoms, but common signs to look out for include:

- few or no periods
- excess hair on the face or breasts, insides of the legs or around the nipples
- acne
- oily skin
- thinning or loss of scalp hair (male-pattern baldness)
- skin tags (known as acrochordons)
- skin discolouration (known as acanthosis nigricans), where the skin looks 'dirty' on the arms, around the neck and under the breasts
- mood swings
- depression
- lack of sex drive
- weight gain, especially around the middle of the body
- difficulty in losing weight
- cravings and binges
- irregular or no ovulation
- difficulty in becoming pregnant
- recurrent miscarriages.

If you have already been diagnosed with PCOS, many of these symptoms will seem horribly familiar. If you haven't been given a diagnosis and you are bothered by any of the above, you should make an appointment to see your GP.

Even if you are diagnosed with PCOS, you should be reassured that many women with polycystic ovaries enjoy regular monthly cycles and have no problem at all getting pregnant. A PCOS diagnosis is only a problem if you also have the hormonal imbalances that cause excess hair or acne or if it affects your menstrual cycle (see pages 14–15).

SYMPTOMS AND THEIR LINK WITH PCOS

Symptom	Percentage with PCOS
Irregular periods	90 per cent
No periods	30–50 per cent
Infertility caused by not ovulating	90 per cent
Acne	95 per cent
Excess hair (hirsutism)	95 per cent

THE CAUSES OF PCOS

Unfortunately, doctors don't yet know what causes PCOS. Some experts believe the problem lies with the ovaries not producing the correct balance of hormones, others hold that the symptoms are triggered in women who produce much too much of a hormone called 'luteinizing hormone' (LH), while others still maintain that PCOS strikes women because they are overweight, or because they seem to have unnaturally high levels of insulin. One theory is that female babies exposed to excess male hormones while inside the womb could be more likely to develop PCOS as adults.[1] There are, however, exceptions to many of these theories: you can be slim and have PCOS, and you can have all the PCOS symptoms, but low levels of LH.

Whatever the explanation, experts have found a possible genetic connection – the condition is known to run in families – and numerous studies show that diet and lifestyle are important. An unhealthy diet and lack of exercise could be enough, in some cases, to push women into developing PCOS, if there is a family susceptibility lurking in the background; or perhaps the only reason PCOS runs in families is because family members eat and behave in the same (unhealthy) way that stimulates PCOS. There is also a theory that in some women PCOS lies dormant, never appearing unless triggered by an unhealthy diet and poor lifestyle with little exercise.

In my opinion, there is probably no one cause for PCOS. It is most likely to be a combination of factors that come together at the same time.

I have found – over and over again – that by treating PCOS as a multi-factorial condition, and addressing as many of the factors as possible at the same time, you can improve the condition considerably. On many occasions I have even seen PCOS reverse completely.

HOW PCOS DEVELOPS

In a normal healthy menstrual cycle, several follicles develop on the surfaces of the ovaries each month. In one of those follicles, a single egg will mature more quickly than the others and be released into the Fallopian tube (sometimes two eggs are released and, if fertilized, will result in twins). The remaining follicles then disintegrate away naturally. But with PCOS, the undeveloped follicles tend to remain on the surface of the ovaries, making them appear enlarged when scanned.

This distortion of the ovary is the most common outward sign of PCOS, but it is merely one of a sequence of hormonal irregularities. The word 'hormone' comes from the Greek 'hormon' and means 'urging on'. Your hormones are the chemical messengers that trigger specific activity in glands and organs of your body, and it is glitches with these messengers that cause the sometimes debilitating symptoms of the condition.

The main function of a healthy menstrual cycle is for one of your ovaries to release a mature egg ready for fertilization. It sounds simple,

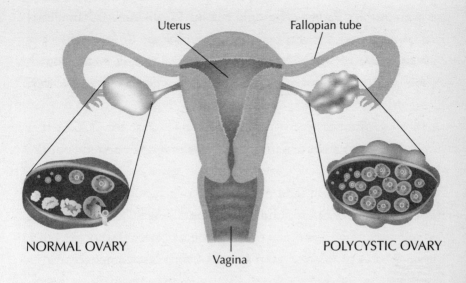

NORMAL OVARY   Vagina   POLYCYSTIC OVARY

but the process requires a number of glands and hormones to be precisely synchronized and the smallest change can throw the whole system out of balance. And that's what PCOS does.

It is a bit like the thermostat on your central heating system. Information about the temperature in the house is fed back to the thermostat and adjustments are made based on that feedback, the boiler going on or off accordingly, so regulating the temperature. But if any part of that feedback loop malfunctions (say the thermostat registers the wrong temperature) the whole system will falter.

Similarly, PCOS creates a destructive vicious cycle of hormonal imbalance which has huge knock-on effects throughout the rest of the body.

With PCOS, the problem often starts with the ovaries, which are unable to produce the hormones they should, and in the correct proportions. But linked to this is the very common problem of a condition called insulin resistance. Insulin is produced by the pancreas to regulate blood sugar. It should help move glucose from the blood after a meal into the muscles to give you energy. But if you develop insulin resistance, your cells can't respond to insulin as they should (they become resistant). Women with PCOS very often have such difficulties with blood-sugar levels, and this too can exacerbate hormonal imbalances.

Inflammation plays a large and sometimes destructive role too. This is not the hot, swollen inflammation you get when you've sprained your ankle or have an infection from a splinter, but a specific process that goes on within the body of someone with PCOS. It is just the body trying to do its utmost to heal itself when PCOS has thrown so many delicate processes out of kilter. It sends out chemicals to try to correct all the imbalances, but, frustratingly, these chemicals very often disrupt the balance even further.

YOUR MENSTRUAL CYCLE

This is what is supposed to happen in a normal menstrual cycle:

1. On the first day of the menstrual cycle, the pituitary gland at the base of the brain releases follicle-stimulating hormone (FSH), which stimulates the ovaries to mature one of their eggs in a follicle and, at the same time, to produce oestrogen.
2. As oestrogen levels increase, FSH levels drop and the pituitary gland releases a surge of LH (luteinizing hormone), which triggers the now mature follicle to release the egg (this is ovulation).
3. The egg is released and the now empty follicle becomes the 'corpus luteum', which produces the hormone progesterone that the body needs to maintain the pregnancy if the egg is fertilized.
4. If the egg is not fertilized, the womb lining (endometrium) breaks away, and that manifests as bleeding, which we know

as a period, and levels of both oestrogen and progesterone fall back into equilibrium once more.

This is what happens during a menstrual cycle when you have PCOS:

1. If you have PCOS, you probably don't have a menstrual cycle or, if you do, it may be irregular with very long gaps in between. FSH is low in relation to LH and the ovaries do not mature a follicle.
2. The complications of PCOS mean that you typically have continually high levels of LH and no discernible surge of LH to trigger ovulation. This means ovulation is less likely to occur and the follicle remains on the surface of the ovary.
3. No egg is released, and there's no 'corpus luteum' to produce progesterone.
4. You may have a period, even if ovulation doesn't happen, but when the pituitary gland registers a lack of progesterone it rightly assumes ovulation hasn't happened and so produces more LH to try to stimulate the follicle to release the egg. This high level of LH triggers the body to produce the male hormone, testosterone, which, ironically, prevents ovulation and causes the creation of those small, multiple follicles on your ovaries. It is these high levels of testosterone that cause the unpleasant PCOS symptoms of excess hair (particularly on the face), thinning hair on the head and acne.

THE ROLE OF INSULIN

Adding to the confused hormone cocktail is the fact that the majority of women with PCOS also suffer from some degree of insulin resistance (see page 16). The insulin receptors on cells are like little locks that need a key (insulin) to open them. So when the receptors are resistant to insulin, the key won't work, the lock can't be opened and

INSULIN RESISTANCE – THE SIGNS

- Tired all the time
- Increased appetite
- Cravings for chocolate, bread, cakes, caffeine and alcohol
- Tendency to gain weight especially around the middle
- Energy slump in the afternoon, needing a bar of chocolate or something to keep you going
- Wanting to eat something sweet after a good meal
- Feeling sleepy after eating
- Eating during the night
- Not sleeping well – can be waking at 3 or 4am
- Brain fog – not thinking clearly and difficulty concentrating

the cell and insulin can't bind together to move the glucose from your blood to use as energy.

Some women inherit a genetic predisposition to becoming insulin resistant. This doesn't mean to say that you will, just that you are more likely to become insulin resistant than the rest of the population and therefore more likely to develop PCOS.

For many women with PCOS, problems with insulin only arise if they eat a lot of refined food (white flour and sugar). Our bodies haven't evolved to function very well on a modern diet of refined foods which are digested too fast and too easily, causing quick spikes in blood-sugar levels. This stimulates the body to produce insulin far more frequently than it should. The result – after years of poor diet – is the insulin overload that causes the cells to become insulin resistant.

Unfortunately, insulin resistance doesn't stop insulin from doing its other job – fat storing. It happily ensures that any glucose in the blood is diverted to the liver, where it is converted into fat and transported in the bloodstream to be stored throughout the body. This process can lead to very difficult-to-shift weight gain and obesity.

If you have PCOS, and you are battling with your weight, it may be comforting to understand that yours is highly likely to be a metabolic problem and that this is why the weight will be harder to shift than it is for most people. But you can do it!

Because an insulin-resistant body cannot use insulin effectively, it will typically ask the pancreas to pump out more and more of it all the time as it attempts to get blood glucose converted into energy. But as insulin levels rise further, there is an unwanted side effect – the excess insulin can stimulate the ovaries to produce yet more testosterone.

The high levels of insulin also stimulate your adrenal glands to produce other male hormones and stimulate the pituitary gland to produce yet more LH.

Another damaging effect of excess insulin is that it causes a drop in production of a specific protein called sex-hormone-binding globulin (SHBG).

Normally, this protein works hard to 'bind' sex hormones like testosterone (bundling them up so they can be shipped out of the system without causing any trouble) and, in so doing, exerts some sort of control over hormone levels circulating in the blood. But high levels of insulin mean low levels of SHBG, which can lead to uncontrolled levels of testosterone.

TESTOSTERONE

All women produce testosterone and all men produce oestrogen – but the quantities vary. Men typically have ten times more testosterone in their systems than women, but women's levels don't have to be particularly high to start seeing negative effects.

THE VICIOUS CIRCLE

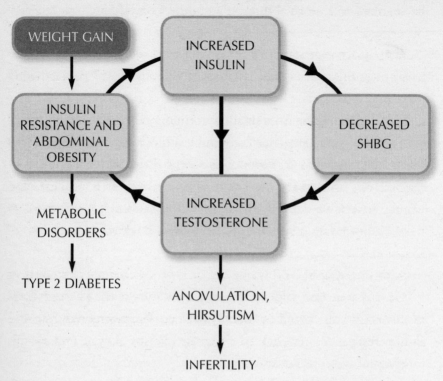

WHY BODY WEIGHT IS IMPORTANT

Many women with PCOS end up overweight. Insulin resistance certainly plays a part, and overweight women are more likely than others to have insulin resistance. Although being overweight does not cause PCOS, it certainly seems to make things worse. Studies show that overweight women with PCOS have higher levels of testosterone, so their 'male' symptoms of excess hair and acne can be more severe.

Also, because the female hormone, oestrogen, is stored in (and to some extent also manufactured by) fat, the more body fat you have, the higher your oestrogen levels are likely to be. The good news is, this means you are less likely to be at risk of problems like osteoporosis (caused by lower levels of oestrogen), but the bad news is you could be at risk of an abnormal thickening of the womb lining (endometrial hyperplasia).

Half of all women with PCOS do not have any problems with their weight, yet they can still have the high LH levels that make the ovaries produce more testosterone. Even if you are not overweight, you may still have higher insulin levels than normal too,[2] and although blood tests may not show that testosterone levels are any higher than they should be, you may experience problems if proportional levels of testosterone and oestrogen are not balanced. This is because slim women have fewer fat cells (to store and manufacture oestrogen), so the male hormones may appear to be dominant (through symptoms of acne and excess hair growth).

Stubborn weight gain is one of the most infuriating symptoms of PCOS, but whatever your weight, if you follow the recommendations in this book you should be able to balance your hormones, improve insulin resistance, get back to a regular menstrual cycle and significantly improve your general health.

STRESS

Stress is known to play a pivotal role in worsening hormonal problems.

When you are under stress your adrenal glands go into overdrive, releasing two hormones: adrenaline and cortisol. Adrenaline ensures you are focused and alert and cortisol increases levels of sugar and fat in your bloodstream, ready for you to run or fight for your life – the fight-or-flight response.

But in the modern world, so many women live their lives under chronic stress, without any break. The resulting constant stream of cortisol increases insulin levels on a continual basis, so stimulating the ovaries to produce yet more testosterone.

Added to all of this is the fact that women also produce male hormones (androgens) from their adrenal glands – they are responsible for about 25 per cent of your circulating testosterone, as well as two other male hormones: androstenedione and DHEAS (dehydroepiandrosterone sulphate).

What all this means is that if you are under stress, you will most likely be producing even more of the male hormones (androgens) that make the skin and hair symptoms of PCOS worse.

THE PCOS VICIOUS CYCLE

With PCOS, everything is linked in a complicated series of connections:

- Too much insulin makes the ovaries produce too much testosterone which affects the development of the follicles in your ovaries.
- When the follicles don't mature properly, you don't ovulate, which makes your body produce too much LH; this, in turn, stops you ovulating.
- LH also stimulates the ovaries to produce too much testosterone.
- Insulin stops your liver from producing the SHBG that mops up excess testosterone and makes your ovaries produce yet more testosterone, which further prevents them from functioning properly.
- The increase in testosterone production exacerbates the insulin resistance, leading to more weight gain, which makes you even more insulin resistant.

When you understand this vicious cycle, and the way in which each part is connected, you will see how it might be possible, bit by bit, to

CULTURAL DIFFERENCES

PCOS affects women all over the world. Scientists have looked at the varying severity of the condition among different cultures in an effort to get a better understanding of it, and interesting distinctions have been found.

Japanese women seem to have fewer problems with excess hair than Italian and US Caucasians, despite similar levels of male hormones. Furthermore, they are rarely overweight, but have similar problems with insulin resistance to Caucasian women.[3]

We know that the incidence of insulin resistance is higher in Mexican–American women with PCOS than native white women, but they have similar testosterone levels,[4] whereas South Asian women develop PCOS at a younger age and have more problems with infertility, insulin resistance and lower SHBG than white women.[5]

break it. In the coming chapters, I will show you how to reset the delicate balance of hormones and get yourself back to good general health.

PCOS AND THE PILL

The Pill has become one of the first drugs doctors reach for when treating PCOS, but all my years of working with sufferers and hearing their stories lead me to suspect that – paradoxically – the contraceptive Pill could itself trigger PCOS symptoms in some women.

The Pill works by suppressing ovulation, making the lining of the womb too thin for implantation and causing the cervical mucus to block the passage of sperm. In suppressing ovulation, it stops the ovary from releasing the egg and renders the ovaries effectively dormant.

Studies show that many women find it takes a long time for ovulation to kick in after stopping the Pill and, very often, conception can be delayed.[6] Certainly, the Pill causes the ovaries to have the appearance of PCOS when seen under an ultrasound scan.

Some experts query the use of the Pill as the standard treatment for PCOS, and questions are being asked as to whether it could actually worsen the problem. One respected study calls for greater research into the long-term effects of oral contraceptives.[7]

This may still be a controversial view, but I believe there could be some groups of women who are so sensitive to the ovarian suppression from the Pill that their ovaries remain inactive when the chemical contraception is removed. It is certainly possible that this inactivity could set up a domino effect throughout the body, triggering all the harmful hormone changes that we associate with PCOS, so I would not recommend using the Pill to treat it.

LONG-TERM HEALTH EFFECTS

If you read this book, and take the steps I recommend, you will certainly notice a reduction in your symptoms and a return to a more normal, balanced state of health. But it is important for you to realize that the lifestyle changes you make now will also have a very significant long-term impact on your health in general.

You may feel that your current PCOS symptoms are bad enough, but unfortunately, statistics show that women with PCOS are seven times more likely to go on to develop Type 2 diabetes because of the problems associated with insulin resistance. They are also at greater risk of heart disease, high blood pressure and stroke (see page 201). And because they may be having fewer (or no) periods, there is an increased risk of the womb lining building up, possibly leading to complications such as endometrial (womb) cancer.

The very good news, however, is that if you follow my recommendations and get your hormones back into healthy balance, you will not only see the symptoms of PCOS diminish but will also be doing the most you possibly can to change your underlying physiology in the long term, benefiting your physical health and, by extension, your mind, and every aspect of how you think and feel.

CHAPTER 2

DIAGNOSING PCOS

Unfortunately, there is still no medical consensus on the criteria for diagnosing PCOS, although it is widely accepted that you should have at least two out of these three problems:

- Infrequent or no ovulation.
- Signs of high levels of male hormones, manifesting either in physical appearance – through hirsutism or acne – or blood tests.
- Polycystic ovaries as seen on an ultrasound scan.

However, if you are bothered by any of the symptoms I describe in Chapter 1 – particularly if you have irregular or no periods or are suffering from infertility, excess hair or acne – I strongly recommend that you talk to your doctor and ask for some tests. (For fuller details on the different criteria used to make a diagnosis of PCOS, see Appendix I, page 209.)

TESTS FOR PCOS

There are a number of tests that help to confirm a diagnosis of PCOS, and because symptoms will vary hugely from woman to woman, you should try to get as many of these as possible. When you know exactly where your hormones are out of balance it becomes so much easier to target the specific nutritional and natural remedies needed to address the problem.

BLOOD TESTS

Normally, your GP will offer a blood test to measure:

- LH (luteinizing hormone) – the hormone that normally triggers ovulation and is often high when you have PCOS
- FSH (follicle-stimulating hormone) – this normally stimulates the ovaries to mature an egg
- testosterone – normally high with PCOS
- free androgen index (FAI) – another measure of male hormone levels
- prolactin (a hormone produced by the pituitary glands – high levels can stop periods)
- fasting glucose – to assess insulin resistance
- thyroid function (TSH – thyroid-stimulating hormone) – to discount the possibility of thyroid problems.

There are a number of other blood tests that might be useful, especially when it comes to focusing on the nutritional recommendations for women with PCOS:

- AMH (anti-mullerian hormone) – this is produced by the ovaries to help the eggs mature each month, and is usually high in women with PCOS (see box, page 29).
- SHBG (sex-hormone-binding globulin) – this works to control levels of sex hormones and is usually low in people with PCOS.
- Fasting insulin – this gives an indication of possible insulin resistance (see page 15).

- Glucose tolerance test – this tests for diabetes.
- Lipid profile – this includes total cholesterol, HDL ('good' cholesterol), LDL ('bad' cholesterol) and triglycerides because PCOS can cause higher levels of total cholesterol and LDL cholesterol.
- DHEAS (dehydroepiandrosterone sulphate) and androstene-dione – both male hormones – and 17-OH progesterone which are all secreted by the adrenal glands or ovaries. Measuring 17-OH progesterone can rule out a condition called congenital adrenal hyperplasia.

Your doctor may or may not tell you the specific results of your blood tests, but if you do ask to see the figures you can get some idea of how out of balance you are by comparing them with the 'normal range' statistics below. If your figures are outside these ranges, but your doctor says you do not have PCOS, you should ask to be referred to a gynaecologist:

Test	Normal range
LH	2–10 iu/l
FSH	2–8 iu/l
AMH	28.6 – 48.5 pmol/l
SHBG	16–119 nmol/l
Testosterone	0.5–3.5 nmol/l
Free androgen index	Less than 5
Prolactin	Less than 500 mU/l
Fasting insulin	Less than 30 mU/l
Fasting glucose	Less than 7 µmol/l
TSH	0.5–5 iu/l

If there is a possibility you may be suffering from PCOS, then the more tests you have the better. With a full set of results at least you know that everything is covered, and your GP or gynaecologist can rule out any other possible causes for your symptoms.

In my opinion, these are the most important tests:

- LH
- FSH
- Testosterone
- Fasting glucose (if you are overweight)

If these results indicate that you might have PCOS your doctor should refer you to a gynaecologist for in-depth blood testing and an ultra-sound scan.

Timing the blood test

If you do have a menstrual cycle (even if it is irregular), you should be tested for FSH and LH on days one to three of your cycle (within the first three days of your period). FSH and LH levels normally increase as the cycle continues, so you need to know your levels at the start of the cycle when they should be at their lowest.

If you are on the contraceptive Pill, your GP won't offer you blood tests for FSH and LH, or even an ultrasound scan to screen for PCOS, because the effects of the Pill on your hormones will very often give misleading results. For an accurate diagnosis, I would advise coming off the Pill and waiting a couple of months before having the test to give your body a chance to start ovulating again, as it can sometimes take a while to do so (if it does at all).

ULTRASOUND SCAN

All women exhibiting PCOS symptoms should be offered an ultra-sound scan so that a proper assessment of the ovaries can be made.

AMH AND FERTILITY TREATMENT

The AMH test is normally used to assess your 'ovarian reserve' (how many eggs you have in storage). This is a useful test to have if you are about to undergo IVF treatment because the lower your AMH levels, the more likely it is that you will respond poorly to IVF drugs.[1]

Very often, if you have PCOS, you will have very high levels of AMH because your smaller PCOS-affected follicles tend to produce more AMH than large follicles.

If you are given IVF treatment (see page 179) you should know that you may be at risk of the fertility drugs over-stimulating your ovaries and so the dose of the fertility medication may need to be reduced. Alternatively, you may be offered another assisted conception technique such as IVM (see page 181) instead of IVF.

This can be performed on the abdomen (just like a pregnancy scan), but a more accurate picture is obtained when the probe is inserted into the vagina. You will be diagnosed with PCOS if the scan shows twelve or more follicles on the ovaries measuring 2–9mm in diameter (the normal size for a healthy follicle is 20mm) and/or increased ovarian volume (more than 10cm³).

OTHER REASONS FOR PCOS SYMPTOMS

Occasionally, PCOS symptoms can be caused by other medical conditions and there are tests that can sometimes be useful in ruling these out.

TSH

Testing for levels of TSH (thyroid-stimulating hormone) will help to rule out thyroid problems by detecting whether your thyroid gland is either overactive (hyperthyroidism) or underactive (hypothyroidism). If the results show your levels of TSH are outside the normal range, you are very likely to be offered further tests.

PROLACTIN

High levels of prolactin indicate possible problems with the pituitary gland (you may be referred for an MRI scan to double check).

LH AND FSH

As we've seen, if you have PCOS, LH levels will normally be high and FSH levels low, but high FSH levels can also be an indicator of early menopause.

CORTISOL

If all your other tests come up negative for PCOS, your doctor may offer you a urine test or bedtime saliva test to measure levels of the stress hormone, cortisol. High levels of cortisol can show that the adrenal glands are over-functioning, and can be indicative of Cushing's syndrome which has many of the same symptoms as PCOS (irregular periods, weight gain – especially around the middle of the body – and insulin resistance).

17-OH PROGESTERONE

The measurement of this hormone can help to rule out adrenal tumours and inherited disorders of the adrenal gland.

CHAPTER 3

YOUR MEDICAL OPTIONS

If your doctor or a gynaecologist diagnoses you with PCOS, you are very likely to be offered any one of a number of drug-based or surgical options to reduce the severity of your symptoms.

It is important that you understand the medical treatments that are available, how they work and the effect they aim to achieve, so that you can make an informed decision about whether or not to go down that route. I do have reservations where these are concerned, since all drugs have side effects and most will merely mask the symptoms of PCOS (which, admittedly, does make life easier), but won't change what is happening to your body. So as soon as you stop taking them, your PCOS symptoms are likely to return.

As a nutritionist, my fundamental aim is to tackle the *cause* of the problem, not merely hide or subdue the symptoms. With my natural approach to PCOS, I've seen symptoms subside time after time, and have even seen the condition disappear completely – with no intervention from drugs or surgery.

Having said that, there's no doubt that drugs and even surgery can help get women through acute and distressing phases of PCOS, particularly when fertility is an issue, but my aim is always to encourage patients to avoid having to take drugs long term, and instead do whatever they can to regulate their hormones in a more natural way.

If you have already been receiving treatment for PCOS, you may be intrigued about the possibility of switching to a more natural approach, or perhaps boosting the impact of your drug treatment by making a few changes to your lifestyle alongside it. For instance, if you choose (or have already been offered) a medical approach, then it's a great idea also to follow my dietary recommendations in Chapter 4, as this integrated line of attack can be very effective.

If you're right at the start of your PCOS journey, and not sure which solutions to choose, my recommendation would always be to read this chapter carefully, and try the nutritional recommendations (see page 39) for three months before making a decision about either drugs or surgery.

PCOS-BUSTING DRUG TREATMENTS

There are a number of drugs that can be used in the treatment of PCOS, each with their own benefits as well as possible side effects. Your doctor will make a choice as to what is best for you but I will describe how they work below so you know exactly what is being offered.

THE CONTRACEPTIVE PILL

A low-dose contraceptive Pill is often suggested to give you regular (but artificial) cycles. It is certainly effective at stopping your womb lining building up abnormally and also helps to increase levels of the protein SHBG, which controls the testosterone freely circulating in your blood. This can contribute to reducing the symptoms of acne and excess hair growth that many PCOS sufferers find so distressing.

The most common brand of Pill offered is Dianette (also known as Diane in many countries) because it contains an anti-androgen progestogen, which can aid in tackling acne and body hair. As already stated, however, every drug has side effects and this one is no different. Studies have shown that Dianette can actually worsen insulin resistance and increase blood levels of insulin[1] (and it carries a greater risk of deep-vein thrombosis than other brands).

Another brand of contraceptive Pill, Yasmin, might be worth considering as it has a diuretic effect, which can reduce water retention and breast tenderness and also acts as an anti-androgen.

You may be offered any number of different brands just to give you a 'regular' cycle and if you do opt for that route, you should ask for one that will help counteract the high levels of male hormones in your system.

While the Pill certainly has a role to play in the short-term treatment of PCOS, my biggest reservation is that it is only useful while you are taking it; if you come off it, your PCOS symptoms inevitably return. Furthermore, I believe the Pill can upset the delicate balance of beneficial bacteria in the gut (as well as in the vagina), making it tougher to lose weight and keep it off. It can also deplete the body of vital nutrients including the B vitamins and especially folic acid, and it can change the ratio of copper and zinc in your body, leaving you with too little zinc and too much copper (see page 191 for information on Nutritional Tests). Zinc is crucial for the normal functioning of your reproductive system and the balance of your hormones.

If you are on the Pill and want to stay on it, I strongly advise you try my dietary recommendations in Chapter 4 and boost your natural defence against PCOS by taking the suggested vitamins and minerals.

If you want to come off the Pill to try my methods on their own, do tell your doctor, but there is no need for you to wean yourself off. You should simply finish that month's course. Obviously, if you don't want to get pregnant, do consider other forms of contraception as sometimes a change in diet can be enough to get your fertility back on track very quickly.

INSULIN SENSITIZERS

Your doctor or gynaecologist may also – or instead – recommend drugs to control your insulin resistance in an attempt to alleviate PCOS symptoms.

The most common drug prescribed in these cases is metformin, which is usually given to people with Type 2 diabetes. Other similar drugs include piaglitazone.

Common side effects can include diarrhoea, nausea and digestive upsets and some women experience an unpleasant metallic taste in their mouths.

Metformin works by not only resensitizing the body to insulin, but it also reduces the absorption of glucose in the digestive system and lowers the liver's production of glucose. By controlling insulin levels, the drug stops the ovaries from producing excess testosterone (excess insulin would normally trigger the release of extra testosterone), and encourages them to produce a more healthy balance of hormones. This can sometimes be enough to help trigger ovulation.

But does it work for PCOS? Studies show conflicting results, with some implying that metformin may alleviate certain PCOS symptoms and not others. It appears to be not as effective as the Pill at regulating the cycle, but it can help induce ovulation which the Pill cannot.[2]

Metformin may be useful in preventing your insulin resistance from developing into Type 2 diabetes, but studies show that diet and exercise work better.[3] In fact, anyone on metformin should certainly be advised to make dietary changes and add exercise into their lives, as the two in combination have been repeatedly proven to aid weight loss.[4] Other studies show that although adding metformin to a diet and exercise programme can improve insulin resistance and testosterone levels, it won't do anything for the hirsutism or the other hormonal imbalances of PCOS.[5]

Another study showed that metformin was less effective than the Pill in regulating the cycle (as one would expect as the Pill is specifically designed to artificially control the cycle) and reducing male hormone levels, but does reduce fasting insulin levels, which the Pill cannot.

Although women with PCOS are routinely prescribed *either* the Pill *or* metformin, it seems to me that a combination of the two drugs could be more effective at tackling more of the symptoms than either on their own.

Metformin can be useful in helping to control the harmful inflammatory processes that PCOS tends to exacerbate in the body; studies show that women taking it had fewer inflammatory markers and increased insulin sensitivity, but women on the Pill had a slight increase in inflammation and no change in insulin sensitivity.[6] This appears to imply that the Pill could actually increase inflammation in the body, which is not good for PCOS or your general health.

COMBINING METFORMIN AND STATINS

Sometimes PCOS can cause cholesterol levels to rise, and you may be offered cholesterol-busting statins to help counteract this. An advantage of these drugs is that as well as lowering cholesterol by blocking its production from the liver, statins do seem to have an anti-inflammatory effect.[7]

Taking metformin in combination with a statin appears to decrease testosterone levels (and ease PCOS symptoms) more effectively than just taking metformin on its own. It can also bring about a greater decrease of LH, total cholesterol and LDL ('bad' cholesterol) and an increase in HDL ('good' cholesterol).[8]

MY VIEW ON DRUGS

The drugs that are commonly prescribed for women with PCOS clearly have some beneficial effects, and for some women there is no doubt they can be lifesavers. But in my experience drugs never solve the problem. As soon as you stop taking them, your PCOS symptoms will return.

Metformin will aid in reducing insulin resistance (temporarily), but the Pill will only artificially override your hormones (when you are on the Pill, you aren't having 'real' periods). Statins may control how much cholesterol your liver produces, but they can't address the fact that your liver is producing too much cholesterol in the first place.

Furthermore, all drugs have side effects, as we know, and taken together they start to impact on each other. Statins, for instance, can increase the blood levels of hormones from the Pill, making it stronger and increasing the risk of side effects. In combination, you could end up with quite a cocktail, which would put your liver under a lot of pressure.

It is worth knowing that if you do take metformin, it increases your risk of vitamin B12 deficiency,[9] which can cause fatigue, diarrhoea, poor memory, pins and needles, menstrual problems, depression and nerve damage.[10] Your multivitamin should contain vitamin B12, but if you have been on metformin for longer than six months, I would suggest you see your GP for a blood test to check whether you are deficient in B12.

SURGERY

If PCOS is causing a problem with fertility, you may be offered surgery to help you ovulate. In Chapter 11: Your Fertility, I give detailed information on the surgical options available to those trying to conceive (see pages 172–81).

PART TWO

NATURAL SOLUTIONS TO PCOS

CHAPTER 4

THE SEVEN-STEP DIET TO BEAT PCOS

The food we eat has been proven, over and over again, to have a huge effect on our health, and after thirty years of treating women with PCOS I can say with great conviction that the dietary recommendations I make in this chapter really will have a noticeable effect on your PCOS symptoms.

By making a few simple alterations to your diet you will be able not only to reduce the severity of symptoms such as acne, weight gain and hirsutism, but you should, in a matter of months, see your body easing back into a more normal way of functioning, with a monthly cycle and – with luck – an end to all the complications you have had to endure with PCOS.

Drugs can certainly ease the intensity of some of the symptoms of PCOS (see Chapter 3), but I don't feel they ever provide a really good long-term solution. Your doctor may prescribe a cocktail of different pills that may ease some of your symptoms and make you feel better, but one thing is for sure: as soon as you stop taking them, the symptoms will return. Most drugs also have a long list of possible side effects, so you may have to weigh up the relative benefits of taking them against other forms of damage they might cause.

However, my diet and lifestyle suggestions will, I strongly believe, dramatically improve the quality of your life, and may even get rid of your PCOS altogether. Unlike drugs, all my methods are natural, safe and work in harmony with a woman's delicate system. What's more, the many happy patients who go through my doors are testament to the effectiveness of this plan.

Sound nutrition is the foundation of good health and you should never underestimate how powerful it can be. It is the fuel that provides you with the energy to live your life and it gives your body the nutrients it needs to produce your hormones in the correct balance. All the cells in your body require nutrients in order to operate properly and the better the supply of those nutrients, the more healthily your cells and body will function, as numerous studies have shown.[1]

This chapter will focus on everything you *should* eat and drink and everything you'd be advised to avoid. The dietary changes I suggest will require quite a bit of commitment on your part, and you'll have to break old habits and say no to a few favourite foods. But believe me, if you have been blighted by PCOS for many years, these small sacrifices will be worth it!

Most importantly though, I will explain here exactly the impact that each dietary change will have on your body, and precisely *how* it will help to control your PCOS symptoms and reset the hormonal imbalances that have taken over your body. I have seen hundreds of PCOS patients over the years, and I see just how hard it is to stick to a diet when you don't understand *why* you have been asked to make changes.

Even if your doctor has prescribed drugs to ease your PCOS symptoms, and you are keen to continue on these, my dietary suggestions will definitely lend a hand. In fact, you may find that if you are taking an insulin sensitizer (like metformin – see page 34), you may be able to reduce the dose because the dietary changes may cause your body to become more sensitive to insulin naturally. Always talk to your doctor first though.

The following seven steps clearly outline how you should adjust your diet to combat PCOS. If you'd like more information on specific foods rich in certain nutrients however, I have provided an easy-to-use list at the back of the book. See Appendix II on page 213.

THE SEVEN STEPS

The fundamental aim of my nutritional approach to PCOS is to target a number of areas simultaneously, so that you get the maximum effect in the minimum amount of time Here's how:

1. **Switch to unrefined carbohydrates** (eaten with protein) and never go more than three waking hours without food to keep your blood-sugar levels balanced.
2. **Eat oily fish and foods rich in Omega 3 fats** to encourage your body to become more sensitive to insulin, so it can overcome insulin resistance.
3. **Cut out all dairy products** for three months to bring levels of male hormones under control.
4. **Eat more vegetables and pulses** to increase levels of the protein SHBG (sex-hormone-binding globulin) which helps to control those male hormones.
5. **Cut right back on or cut out alcohol** for twelve weeks to allow your liver function to improve.
6. **Cut down on caffeine** to give your adrenal glands a rest.
7. **Cut down on saturated fats and eliminate completely unhealthy trans fats** to counter the potentially damaging inflammatory processes PCOS causes in the body.

1. SWITCH TO UNREFINED CARBOHYDRATES

I believe this step to be the most important dietary change any PCOS sufferer can make, as it constitutes the foundation of all healthy eating. You just need to switch your refined carbohydrates (white bread, pasta, rice, etc.) to unrefined (wholemeal bread and pasta and brown rice). Then you have to ensure you eat little and often, adding protein (vegetable or animal) (see page 45) to each meal, and never allowing yourself to get hungry.

These changes are designed to help your body keep blood-sugar levels in balance.

A diet rich in unrefined carbohydrates is the best way to prevent or reverse the insulin resistance that is at the heart of PCOS, and it is also the best way to ensure you lose weight (if you are one of the many sufferers whose PCOS has caused weight gain).[2]

The reason it works is simple: all carbohydrates (sugars and starches) are broken down by your body into glucose when you eat them, and the faster they are broken down, the more dramatic (and destructive) the effect on your blood-sugar levels – particularly if you have PCOS. A rise in blood-sugar levels triggers the pancreas to release insulin, and the higher the rise, the more insulin has to be released. When a food gets refined, a lot of fibre is discarded along with valuable nutrients, whereas if it is unrefined, the natural fibre remains intact, your body takes longer to break the food down and so it hits your bloodstream more slowly.

Some carbohydrates (sugar, for instance) are broken down very quickly, causing a rush of glucose into the blood, while others (such as brown rice) take longer to metabolize and give the body plenty of time to deal with them before they can do any damage, or start triggering any hormonal reactions. If you switch from sugary, quick-burn foods to slow-burn whole foods, you create steady, slow lifts in blood sugar to which your body hardly has to respond – only having to release a small amount of insulin to deal with them.

Your doctor may have already suggested that you switch to a healthy diet, but numerous studies show that sticking specifically to slow-burn, unrefined foods really does help more.[3]

You can measure the speed at which any food is metabolized by its glycaemic index (GI). A fast-burn food will have a high GI, while a slow-burn food has a low GI. But instead of worrying about the GI value for certain foods (or even getting involved in another measure which calculates each food's 'glycaemic load' or GL) I suggest you simply think of carbohydrates in terms of whether they are refined or unrefined.

Unrefined	Refined
Barley	Biscuits, cakes and pastries made
Brown rice	with white flour and sugar
Buckwheat (part of	Breakfast cereals with added sugar
rhubarb family)	Brown and white sugar
Fruit (particularly berries,	Chocolate
apples and pears and citrus)	Fruit juice (as the fibre has been
Maize	removed)
Millet	Honey
Oats	Instant porridge oats
Rye	Sugar
Spelt	Soft fizzy drinks
Vegetables	Treacle
Wholemeal breads	White flour
Wholemeal flour	White rice
Wholemeal pasta	

FRUIT JUICE

Fruit juice is considered a 'refined carbohydrate' because most of the fibre has been removed. This means the fruit sugar (fructose) hits your bloodstream quickly, forcing your body to release a lot of insulin to deal with that quick surge. You should limit your intake of fruit juice if you are trying to control your insulin levels. Whole fruit, with all its fibre intact, is a much better option. In fact, one large long-term study found that increasing fruit and vegetable consumption *reduced* the risk of diabetes, but increasing fruit juice consumption by just one serving a day gave an 18 per cent *increased* risk of diabetes.[4]

So either dilute your fruit juice half and half with water or opt for a smoothie (which contains the fibre from the fruit) instead. Also, avoid anything called 'fruit juice drink', as it may contain sugar or artificial sweeteners.

FIBRE

There are two forms of fibre: soluble (which dissolves in water) and insoluble (which doesn't). Both contribute to a sense of fullness and satisfaction and can help with weight loss.

The insoluble fibre found in whole grains and vegetables keeps your bowels healthy, but the soluble fibre found in oats and beans has been shown to have a very useful impact on controlling blood sugar.[5] Soya and the other legumes like chickpeas and lentils contain both soluble and insoluble fibres and research has shown that soya can decrease insulin resistance.[6] (The benefits of soya and the other legumes in boosting SHBG are discussed on page 55).

Adding protein

You can improve the effect of your unrefined carbohydrates even further if you try to include protein in every meal and most snacks. So, whenever you eat an oat cake, or a piece of wholemeal bread, try to include a little bit of fish or egg or a vegetable protein such as quinoa, legumes (hummus), nuts (nut butters are good, e.g. almond butter) or seeds. The body takes longer to process proteins than other foods, so by adding protein to a meal you effectively slow down the absorption, allowing the carbohydrate to hit the bloodstream in a steady trickle, rather than a quick hit.

The great beauty of the PCOS way of eating is that it is not a calorie-counting diet, or even, specifically, a weight-loss diet. The key issue is the effect of the food you choose on your body and insulin levels. Having said that, after a few weeks of eating like this, you will not only feel so much better, you will, in all likelihood, lose weight too.

One reason is because refined foods contain very little goodness (so many nutrients being lost in the refining process), and if you, like so many people, have lived for years on a poor diet of fast food, white bread, sweets and snacks, you could easily end up being deficient in essential nutrients. Your body will typically respond by increasing your

FREE FOODS!

Some foods contain so much fibre in relation to their carbohydrate content that you can eat as much of them as you like without any risk of a high rise in blood glucose and a subsequent high release of insulin. Examples of these 'free foods' are asparagus, aubergine, beans, broccoli, Brussels sprouts, cabbage, cauliflower, kale (all cooked) and celery, fennel, lettuce, olives, peppers, tomatoes, avocados, raspberries and strawberries (all eaten raw).

appetite to try to get those valuable nutrients from a larger amount of food and by storing fat (because it thinks you are starving). The more refined the food you eat, the more deficient you become and the more your appetite and cravings increase, driving you, in turn, to eat more refined nutritionally deficient food.

Just making the switch to healthy, unrefined food can be enough to stop that vicious circle, and shift weight – without the need for dieting.

SUGAR

It is really crucial to try to cut down on added sugar as much as you possibly can. Sugar is, by definition, one of the most refined of the carbohydrates and a real enemy of women with PCOS.

Sugar is added (without you realizing) to so many foods and most of us consume around forty-six teaspoons of the stuff every day.[7] Cutting back on it can be really tough at first, but once you start eating more healthily, your tastes will naturally change and your body will crave fewer sugary foods. There are also supplements that will assist with this (such as chromium – see page 70).

Sugar comes in many different guises – fructose, glucose, dextrose (made from cornstarch), lactose (milk sugar), maltose, sucrose (common table sugar made from sugar cane or beet), corn syrup (made from corn) – so it's a good idea to get into the habit of reading the labels on foods.

Manufacturers are obliged to list all the ingredients in a food product with the largest ingredient first, so to avoid the word 'sugar' looming large on the label, they mix in smaller amounts of the different types of sugars. This means the sugars can be peppered throughout the ingredients list without you realizing just how much they have added.

Be aware also that sugar is added to savoury foods like tomato ketchup and soups, mayonnaise and salad dressing; and a supposedly healthy fruit yogurt can contain as much as eight teaspoons of added sugar. Watch out for the 'healthy'-looking breakfast cereals, where some can contain more sugar than a doughnut (11.1g/3 teaspoons) in a small bowl of cereal compared to 8.6g in one doughnut).

My advice, particularly for those with PCOS, is to avoid *any* products with added sugar and to try to find a no-sugar alternative. Try a smearing of pure fruit (sugar-free) jam on wholemeal toast, and look out for biscuits sweetened with apple juice – both can be useful in weaning you off added sugar (a small amount of fruit juice used as a sweetener is fine compared to a glass of fruit juice). I don't recommend a switch to artificial sweeteners in order to avoid sugar, as studies show they can confuse the body and don't help you to lose weight.[8] In fact, artificial sweeteners make your body crave other foods and can increase your appetite.

Eat little and often

It is quite clear that *what* you eat can have a huge impact on your PCOS, but also important is the timing of *when* you eat.

To keep blood-sugar levels stable you need to create a slow, low rise in blood sugar after a meal, so your pancreas does not have to produce large amounts of insulin to deal with a quick sugar rush, and you need to try to maintain a steady level until the next meal or snack is eaten.

The trick is to eat little and often and not to allow more than three hours to pass between meals. I recommend breakfast, lunch and dinner with a mid-morning and mid-afternoon snack. Don't skip breakfast. If you do, by 10 or 11am your blood sugar will have dropped so low that your body will be urging you to go for a quick fix (a cup of coffee or a biscuit) to boost it, so there's a little fuel for your poor addled brain.

If you leave long gaps without eating (as so many people do when they're trying to lose weight), your body will think there is a shortage of food and will very cleverly slow down your metabolism, holding tightly on to your fat stores. When you do then finally eat it will – equally cleverly – work really hard to absorb as many calories as possible from that meal because it thinks you might not eat again for a long time.

By making the switch to eating little and often you will be effectively telling your body that there is an abundance of food out there, allowing it to rev up your metabolism so that your body will let go of fat stores. Indeed, research in adolescents has shown that snackers tend to be less overweight and obese and have less fat around the middle (which is common in PCOS).[9]

So eating little and often should ensure you have steady energy levels throughout the day without a mid-afternoon slump, and that you lose your cravings for sweets, chocolate, cakes and sweets. These cravings can be impossible to resist if your blood sugar has dropped so low (hypoglycaemia) that your body urges you to find a quick, high-sugar fix. The brain needs a constant trickle of blood sugar to function, and will react to a drop by either releasing stress hormones which will let sugar loose from the stores or creating an impossible-to-resist craving for you to eat more sugar. This has nothing to do with weak willpower; it is a strong physiological urge designed to correct low blood-sugar levels.

As a bonus, your new eating patterns should help to eradicate any mood swings too, smoothing out the highs and lows and feelings of anxiety, irritability and tension that characterize volatile blood-sugar levels (for more information on stress, see page 129).

2. EAT OILY FISH AND FOODS RICH IN OMEGA 3 FATS

Forget switching to a tasteless, low-fat diet. If you really want to clear your PCOS you need to boost your intake of the sort of healthy fats you find in oily fish such as salmon, nuts and seeds.

These good fats are called 'essential fatty acids' because they are essential to your health. They include the polyunsaturated fats Omega 6 and Omega 3, the most vital of which – for PCOS sufferers – are the Omega 3s. They aid in overcoming insulin resistance and also have a part to play in heart health and the prevention of diabetes, obesity and high blood pressure.[10]

These Omega 3 fats, which so many women hardly include in their diets any more, are crucial for keeping your cell walls flexible. Without an adequate supply of them in the diet, your cell walls harden and their insulin receptors become unresponsive to insulin. This means insulin resistance sets in, triggering all the problems of PCOS.

With healthy fats like Omega 3s in the diet, however, the cell walls become healthier, their insulin receptors become more sensitive to insulin and both willing and able to take the sugar (glucose) from your blood and use it for energy. If your body is able to use insulin effectively, it no longer has to produce extra-high amounts to get the job done.

The Omega 3 fats also help to reduce male hormones and so can address both acne and excess hair growth.[11]

Omega 3 fats are found in oily fish (such as mackerel, salmon and sardines. If you are vegetarian, you can still get them from flaxseeds (linseeds) or soya, but the levels are lower than they would be in fish.

You'll also get even less goodness from these foods if you are stressed, drinking too much alcohol or not getting enough other key nutrients (particularly zinc, magnesium and vitamin B6). If you are vegetarian you should consider taking Omega 3 fats in supplement form (see page 75).

These days you can buy certain foods – such as some milks and breads – that claim to be fortified with Omega 3s. It seems a good idea, but the quantities can be minimal – you'd have to eat twenty-three slices of bread a day to get sufficient Omega 3 to make a difference. It's probably easier to eat one portion of salmon, herring, sardines or mackerel (fresh, frozen or tinned). Fresh tuna is good too, but sadly much of the Omega 3s are lost in the tuna canning process so tinned tuna isn't so good. Salmon, herring, trout and sardines are the best sources. However, you should not eat too much oily fish, as sea fish can contain heavy metals like mercury and other pollutants such as dioxins and PCBs. (PCBs, or polychlorinated biphenyls, are manmade substances used in industry. Although they are no longer produced in the UK and US they cannot be broken down and so they persist in the environment as a pollutant.) These toxins are stored in fat, and because oily fish are, by definition, fattier than white fish, they potentially contain more of the pollutants. It's a good idea to restrict yourself to four portions per week (two if you're pregnant or trying to conceive) and keep fish like marlin and swordfish to occasional treats as these tend to live longer lives, making them more likely to have accumulated mercury levels in their fat. And because the Omega 3 fats are so important for PCOS, I suggest you take some in supplement form too (see page 75). The good supplements are screened for heavy metals like mercury and also dioxins, so you know they are safe.

Not only do Omega 3 fats help your body overcome insulin resistance, but studies show that Omega 3 supplements can contribute to reducing testosterone levels in women with PCOS.[12]

3. CUT OUT ALL DAIRY PRODUCTS

Milk, cheese and butter contain a substance called insulin-like growth factor (IGF-1), which is similar in structure to insulin. Its insulin-like properties mean it can stimulate the storage of glucose in fat cells, and can trigger increased production of testosterone.

We all produce a certain amount of IGF-1 in our bodies, with levels peaking in puberty (when we tend to get acne), but usually declining

CINNAMON AS A NATURAL INSULIN SENSITIZER

Try sprinkling a teaspoon of cinnamon on your porridge or in a herbal tea each day. Studies show the spice can be active in reducing blood glucose levels and improve insulin resistance in those with Type 2 diabetes.[13] It has also been shown to help improve insulin sensitivity in women with PCOS.[14]

Cinnamon could also play a role in the long-term prevention of insulin resistance, metabolic syndrome and Type 2 diabetes as studies show it has beneficial effects on insulin, insulin sensitivity and body-fat composition.[15]

Warning: do not consume large amounts of cinnamon if you have a bleeding disorder or if you are taking a blood thinner, such as heparin or warfarin, as it contains a substance called coumarin, which can have a blood-thinning effect.

as we get older. However, tests have shown that women with PCOS can have twice as much IGF-1 in their bodies as other women,[16] and that the ovaries of women with PCOS are more sensitive to IGF-1.[17]

IGF-1 is involved in the maturing of the follicles on the ovary and stimulates the production of male hormones from the ovaries, increasing androgen production from the adrenal glands. It specifically stimulates an enzyme called 5 alpha reductase, which converts testosterone to its stronger form DHT (dihydrotestosterone), causing acne and hirsutism in people with PCOS.

If you are affected by acne and excess hair, it makes a lot of sense to try to reduce IGF-1 in your diet. Milk could be the biggest culprit. Because of modern farming methods, milk today seems to have far higher levels of IGF-1 than ever before, so it makes sense to cut out dairy products, and switch to rice milk or soya milk instead. This

DAIRY FOODS AND CALCIUM INTAKE

Dairy foods have long been touted as an important source of calcium. But many cultures around the world live quite healthily without them in their diet.

An adult needs about 700mg of calcium a day and it is easy to make this up with other non-dairy foods:

Food (3½oz/100g portion)		Calcium (mg)
Fish	Pilchards in tomato sauce	250
	Sardines in tomato sauce	430
	Sardines in oil	500
	Whitebait, fried	860
	Salmon, tinned	91
	Tuna in oil, tinned	12
Vegetables	Curly kale, boiled	150
	Okra, stir-fried	220
	Spring greens, boiled	75
	Watercress	170
Pulses, beans and seeds	Red kidney beans	71
	Tofu, steamed*	510
	Green/French beans	56
	Baked beans	53
	Sesame seeds	670
	Tahini (sesame paste)	680
Cereal products	Wholemeal bread	106
	Muesli, Swiss-style	110

Fruit		
	Apricots, dried	73
	Figs, dried	250
	Currants	93
	Mixed peel	130
	Olives, in brine	61
	Orange	47

* Different products vary considerably
(Table taken from McCance and Widdowson's 'The Composition of Foods' Sixth Summary Edition 2002. Compiled by the Food Standards Agency and Institute of Food Research.)

If you are worried you might be lacking in calcium you can always add a multivitamin and mineral containing calcium (see Chapter 5 for advice on supplements).

doesn't have to be a permanent measure, but I'd recommend you keep off milk for at least one month, ideally three, so you can see whether there's any change to your PCOS symptoms.

Alongside exercise, cutting out dairy has been shown to have a beneficial effect on controlling the production of male hormones that can make PCOS so distressing.[18]

The other interesting thing about milk is although it has a low GI (so it shouldn't cause rapid spikes in blood-sugar levels), it can cause a high level of insulin to be secreted[19] – if you add just 200ml milk to a low-GI meal it causes an increase in insulin response of 300 per cent, thereby transforming it into a very high-GI meal.[20]

Other research has shown that drinking one glass of milk a day can increase your risk of ovarian cancer.[21] Scientists believe this could be something to do with the milk sugar lactose, but it could be down to a combination of the lactose and IGF-1 (see page 50). If milk can increase your risk of ovarian cancer, it could have a negative effect on your ovaries, so I really think it's a good idea to cut out milk if you have PCOS and are trying to get and keep your ovaries functioning normally.

If you have already switched to unrefined carbohydrates (Step 1) and you are increasing your intake of healthy fats (Step 2), you will already be part of the way towards controlling the levels of male hormones in your body. The unrefined carbohydrates will be stopping your body from producing too much insulin which would normally be stimulating your ovaries to produce testosterone. Studies show that the lower your natural insulin levels, the more effective your body will be at blocking the harmful action of IGF-1. Following a low GI diet for just twelve weeks is enough to reduce levels of IGF-1 and significantly improve acne.[22]

If you are also sticking to Step 2 of my eating plan, the healthy fats in your diet should mean that your cells are gradually becoming more sensitive to insulin. This should help reduce insulin production and therefore testosterone levels.

These lower levels of insulin should also mean you have more of the crucial protein SHBG (sex-hormone-binding globulin) in your system which binds to (and so helps control levels of) testosterone.

Even if it seems like a bit of an effort to make these changes to your diet, particularly if you've always eaten refined carbohydrates, sugary foods and lots of milk, trust me, the effort will DEFINITELY be worth it. You will already be making very positive changes in your hormone balance, your PCOS symptoms, your fertility and your long-term health.

If you really do want to include a little dairy in your diet I recommend you choose organic products as they tend to contain a better balance of beneficial fats. Levels of Omega 3 in organic milk can be up to 60 per cent higher than in non-organic and up to 40 per cent lower in saturated fat, even though the total fat content is the same.[23] This

THE SEVEN-STEP DIET TO BEAT PCOS

is probably because organic cows eat grass rather than processed food and this changes the fat composition of the milk. For the same reason, I'd always choose organic butter over margarine as I think it is a more natural product.

4. EAT MORE VEGETABLES AND PULSES

Your liver produces SHBG (sex-hormone-binding globulin) – a clever protein which latches on to excess hormones like testosterone in your blood and stops them from circulating freely. When you've got PCOS, your SHBG levels are very likely to be extremely low, which just makes symptoms like acne and hirsutism worse. However, if you up your daily intake of vegetables, you can hugely boost levels of this highly beneficial protein in your blood.

We know that raised insulin levels keep SHBG production low, so by following the dietary steps in this chapter in general, you should be getting your blood sugar under control, so reducing your need for excess insulin and allowing SHBG levels to lift once more. However, studies show that, in particular, the more vegetables you eat, the higher your SHBG levels will be,[24] and also that a higher intake of lignans – found in flaxseeds (linseeds) – is associated with a higher level of SHBG and a lower level of testosterone.[25]

So vegetables really are crucial here. SHBG levels have been shown to be 23 per cent lower in women who eat a lot of meat and starchy foods, but much higher in those whose diets are rich in vegetables and pulses such as soya, chickpeas and lentils.[26]

As an added complication, studies have shown that women with PCOS who record low levels of SHBG could also be at risk of a condition called metabolic syndrome (which, in turn, carries an increased risk of heart disease, high blood pressure, diabetes and cancer).[27] This can clearly affect long-term health.

So if by upping your intake of vegetables and pulses you can reduce testosterone levels in your system, ease the PCOS symptoms of acne and excess hair, *and* be healthier in the long term, it's clearly a great dietary step to take.

5. CUT RIGHT BACK ON OR CUT OUT ALCOHOL

Your liver plays a significant part in the balance of blood sugar and in detoxifying and eliminating hormones. If you really do want to control your PCOS, you need to give your liver a break from the rigours of trying to metabolize alcohol, so it can concentrate more fully on helping sort out your PCOS symptoms. I therefore recommend that all my PCOS patients eliminate alcohol completely for twelve weeks or, at the very least, cut back to the absolute minimum of one to two units over a weekend only – one unit of alcohol being a small glass of wine, half a pint of beer or a single measure of spirits. But this is only an approximate guide as a unit depends on the percentage of alcohol in the drink and the higher the alcohol content of the drink, the less units you can safely drink because it is stronger.

The liver is the largest organ in your body and has many functions including the storage and filtration of blood, conversion of sugars into glycogen, the metabolism of fat and the ability to use it to produce energy. It is also your waste-disposal unit for drugs, alcohol, toxins, pollutants and, specifically, your hormones, and is where the important protein SHBG is produced (see page 55).

The health of your liver and its smooth functioning are so critical when you are trying to sort out your PCOS that I cannot emphasize enough the significance of giving it a bit of a rest so it can do its job to the best of its ability.

When you drink alcohol it will be absorbed into the bloodstream very quickly and rushed to the liver. However, your liver cannot store alcohol, so it has to break it down to eliminate it. The more you drink in one session, the harder your liver has to work. A healthy liver can deal with about one unit an hour, so if you drink more than one unit in that time period, your liver has to store it as fat in the liver, which can cause fatty liver disease. The breakdown product of the alcohol, acetaldehyde, can also cause your arteries to narrow, increasing the risk of heart disease.

If that wasn't enough, alcohol can lead to more weight gain around the middle of your body, which, because tummy fat is metabolically active, can increase the severity of your PCOS symptoms.

Alcohol is classed as an anti-nutrient, which means that it can block the absorption of really useful nutrients like zinc (which is crucial for hormone regulation) from your food. It is also a diuretic so you can end up losing even more nutrients through your urine.

Red wine

Research shows that red wine in moderation can be beneficial and even reduce the risk of heart disease.[28] Red wine contains an antioxidant called resveratrol, which helps to increase a hormone called adiponectin; this is involved in making your body more sensitive to insulin and aids in protecting the heart.

But before you reach for the Cabernet Sauvignon, you should know resveratrol is found in the grapes and you can also take it as a supplement.

IMPROVE LIVER FUNCTION

Onions, leeks and garlic contain sulphur compounds which can assist liver function, while vegetables of the cruciferous family (broccoli, Brussels sprouts, cauliflower and cabbage) help the liver to detoxify oestrogen. Artichoke and dandelion greens are great to eat too, as they support your liver in producing bile which breaks fats down into small molecules so that they can be digested more easily.

6. CUT DOWN ON CAFFEINE

If you have, by now, made the switch to unrefined carbohydrates, you will already be working hard to keep your blood-sugar levels on an even keel. It is the energy dips and troughs and long gaps between meals that trigger the adrenal glands into action, encouraging them to pump out the stress hormones that are so harmful for sufferers of PCOS. But if you are serious about getting to the bottom of your PCOS symptoms, you really need to try to keep those adrenal glands as happy as possible.

The key to adrenal health is to cut right back on caffeine. Anything containing caffeine acts as a stimulant that will make your body release more of the stress hormones and cause blood-sugar levels to fluctuate. We know that women with PCOS have increased levels of the stress hormone cortisol,[29] so it is vital to help reduce these in order to reduce insulin levels.

Like alcohol, caffeine also acts as a diuretic, so if you drink a lot, you risk losing valuable nutrients like zinc (which is crucial for hormone balance) through your urine.

Caffeine is found in coffee, tea (black, green and white) and colas, but also chocolate (more so in dark than milk chocolate because the cocoa solids are higher).

Green tea does contain caffeine, but it is healthier for PCOS sufferers than traditional black tea for a number of reasons: it is less processed and fermented and is usually drunk without milk; it contains antioxidants, which are generally beneficial to your health and can help inhibit the growth of cancer cells;[30] and it can assist in lowering cholesterol. Green tea could also contribute to weight loss as it has a mild fat-burning effect.[31]

But the main benefit of green tea in relation to your PCOS is that it is active in detoxification in general, and especially the detoxification of oestrogen,[32] and it could also assist in improving insulin sensitivity.[33]

Although there has been little research into the benefits of white tea, it is less processed than green tea, and is said to contain more of the polyphenol catechins. It these catechins which are thought to be responsible for the cancer-, heart-disease- and diabetes-prevention benefits.

I would suggest you reduce or eliminate your intake of coffee and black tea and substitute the occasional cup of green or white tea instead, adding some herbal teas such as peppermint or chamomile into the mix. I don't recommend decaffeinated coffee because even though the caffeine is removed, other stimulants (theobromine and theophylline) remain and will have some effect on your adrenal glands. Decaffeinated tea is stimulant-free, but will contain residues of the chemicals used to remove the caffeine.

CAFFEINE CONTENT OF DIFFERENT DRINKS (8FL OZ)

Coffee, instant	66mg
Coffee, filtered	120mg
Tea, ordinary black	60mg
Colas	45–50mg
Tea, green	15mg
Tea, white	15mg
Cocoa	14mg
Hot Chocolate, dark (1fl oz)	20mg
Hot Chocolate, milk (1fl oz)	6mg
Coffee, decaffeinated	5mg

Caffeine withdrawal

When you come off caffeine, do so slowly to avoid withdrawal symptoms such as headaches and feeling like you have the flu, with muscle cramps and fatigue. Substitute one cup a day with a decaffeinated alternative, then, when you are only drinking decaffeinated coffee or tea, gradually substitute those, again one cup a day, with herbal tea or even a grain coffee (which is available in health food shops and contains chicory and barley, for example).

7. CUT DOWN ON SATURATED FATS AND ELIMINATE COMPLETELY UNHEALTHY TRANS FATS

Not all fats are equal. There are those – the Omega 3s – that I'm really keen for you to include in your diet and to take additionally as supplements, but there are some that don't help your fight against PCOS and still others that I think you should make every attempt to avoid completely because they have such a negative effect on your health and on your ability to overcome PCOS.

There is a common misconception that polyunsaturated fats like Omega 6 are great for your health. To an extent this is true, and many women swear by huge doses of evening primrose oil (rich in Omega 6) in the fight against PMS problems. But studies show that the really useful work of the meagre Omega 3s we do manage to glean from our modern diets is diminished by the high levels of Omega 6 so many of us consume.

It is estimated that we are getting up to twenty-five times more Omega 6 fats from our diet than Omega 3s and that for good health it should be nearer a ratio of one to one.[34] Many of the women I see in the clinic have been taking evening primrose oil supplements for years and have not been eating enough Omega 3 oils, or taking them in supplement form, to counterbalance this. Some women are also taking combinations such as Omega 3, 6 and 9 in supplement form because they have heard that we need a good balance of all the Omega fats. This is true, but you have to take into account other sources of these fats in your diet. So if you eat a lot of foods containing vegetable oils, your diet is probably very high in Omega 6 already. (You can do a simple home finger-prick blood test to tell if you have the correct balance of Omega 3 to Omega 6 in your body – go to www.natural-healthpractice.com.)

Also, if you have high levels of insulin in your system, as many women with PCOS do, and high levels of Omega 6, the two can react together to produce compounds that increase the destructive inflammatory response in the body.

Your body produces substances called prostaglandins from the Omega 3 and 6 fatty acids, some of which cause inflammation and some of which are anti-inflammatory. The more Omega 6 you have in your body in relation to Omega 3, the more inflammation your body will produce (see below).

My advice is to increase your intake of oily fish and to reduce your intake of Omega 6 by cutting down on polyunsaturated vegetable oils like sunflower and corn oil. Olive oil (Omega 9 oil) is good to use for cooking.

Saturated fats

It's a really good idea for PCOS sufferers to try to reduce their intake of the saturated fats found in meat and dairy products, as well as in tropical oils like coconut (which I will discuss on page 92) and palm oil. High intakes of saturated fats make it more difficult for your body to absorb the Omega 3 fats efficiently which, in turn, leads to an increase of inflammation in your body. Research shows that saturated fats induce inflammatory activity and increase insulin resistance.

Inflammation is something we should all seek to avoid, but it is more pertinent still if you have PCOS. The more inflammation you have in your body, the worse your insulin resistance is likely to become and the more weight you are likely to gain around the middle of your body. This tummy fat is metabolically active and adds to the inflammation process, just making things worse.

Women with PCOS can record inflammation levels that are 96 per cent higher than they should be, even if they are not overweight. We measure inflammation with a blood test for an 'inflammatory marker' called CRP (C Reactive Protein)[35] and tests are available through my clinic (see Useful Resources, page 217).

Doctors now believe the inflammation process is responsible for a whole host of degenerative diseases such as heart disease and cancers, and the more bad fat you have in your diet, and the more fat you accumulate around the middle of your body, the more inflammation you will have. Fat – also called adipose tissue – around the middle is not an inert substance; it is active and functions in its own right, manufacturing and releasing different substances.

Fat cells are also able to produce an immune response in the body, which causes inflammation. In evolutionary terms, this inflammatory response allowed the fat stores to help fight infection by producing substances called inflammatory cytokines, which have the effect of pumping up the immune system. This urges the adrenal glands to release more cortisol to calm it down. However, in most women, the excess cortisol in their system causes more fat to be stored, which then releases more inflammatory cytokines.

Fat cells also secrete oestrogen and two other compounds – tumour necrosis factor alpha and resistin – both of which interfere with the functioning of insulin. Your body will try to compensate by making yet more insulin which, in turn, causes more inflammation and leaves you stuck in a vicious cycle.

Eggs and oily fish also contain some saturated fats, as well as the healthy Omega 3 fats. If you are concerned about saturated fats, you don't need to become vegetarian to avoid them. If you are eating meat or chicken, buy free-range or organic as they are going to contain healthier fats than corn-fed animals because of the balance of fats that metabolizes from the food they eat.

Trans fats

With no nutritional benefits at all, these are the worst fats and should be avoided at all costs.

Found in many processed foods (such as shop-bought cakes, biscuits and fast foods) to prolong their shelf life, they might appear on the label as hydrogenated or partially hydrogenated vegetable oil.

Trans fats are produced by chemically altering liquid oils to make them into solids by passing hydrogen through the oil at a high temperature and under pressure. They act like a plastic, so your body does not know what to do with them, and they can cause all sorts of unhealthy processes to occur.

These fats have been linked to an increased risk of heart disease and are terrible for your general health, but they are particularly bad for you if you have PCOS. Just 4g of trans fats a day has been shown to interfere with ovulation, giving a 73 per cent increase in the risk of ovulatory infertility.[36]

Trans fats will also cause you to put on more weight around the middle of the body, even if you are sticking to a low-calorie diet,[37] and they block the absorption of the essential fatty acids which are needed to overcome insulin resistance and so hinder any attempts you might be making to reverse your insulin sensitivity.

Trans fats harden cells and arteries (which is why they are linked to heart disease), but they can also harden your insulin receptors, making you more insulin resistant and encouraging your body to produce even higher amounts of insulin to overcome the resistance.

Studies show that avoiding trans fats can reduce the risk of diabetes by 40 per cent,[38] so it is extremely important to steer clear of trans fats if you want to try to improve your insulin sensitivity.

Not only do trans fats create more inflammation in the body, but they also block the production of beneficial anti-inflammatory substances, giving them a horrific double negative effect when it comes to trying to control inflammation.

Trans fats have been banned in a number of places (including Denmark, Switzerland, Austria and New York), not only in food products, but also in restaurants and fast-food outlets. According to UK officials, however, a ban would be too difficult to implement, so just be vigilant and read *all* food labels carefully.

HOW TO REDUCE INFLAMMATION

The drug metformin, which is commonly prescribed to women with PCOS (see page 34), is known to help reduce inflammation, but I passionately believe it is healthier to achieve this using foods, supplements and herbs rather than drugs, which can have side effects.

Get some beneficial bacteria

Getting the levels of beneficial bacteria right can actually aid your efforts to lose weight and can play a major role in helping control inflammation.[39] Research has suggested that certain 'negative' bacteria may actually cause inflammation. I would recommend taking probiotics in supplement form, rather than in drink or yogurt form (as outlined in Chapter 5), firstly to make sure you are getting enough of the beneficial bacteria and also because the probiotic drink or yogurt could be loaded with sugar, which is counterproductive to your PCOS health plan.

Enjoy the sunshine!

Vitamin D, which your body manufactures from sunshine, is very useful in helping to control inflammation and it also improves insulin sensitivity.[40]

If you are trying to get pregnant or are having recurrent miscarriages, I'd advise you to get your vitamin D levels checked. Good levels of vitamin D help the body maintain a pregnancy by effectively switching off the part of the immune system that could reject a baby. (You can get a simple home finger-prick test for vitamin D; go to www.naturalhealthpractice.com.)

These days, an increasing number of women could end up deficient in vitamin D without realizing it. In the UK vitamin D levels are alarmingly low, with more than 50 per cent of adults being deficient,[41] while Australians have a 1 in 4 deficiency.[42] You need about thirty minutes' exposure to the sun up to three times a week to produce a healthy level of vitamin D, so make the most of the summer months and consider taking a supplement, too.

There is a wonderful domino effect when you start making my dietary changes. Each small change has a positive knock-on effect on all the different hormonal activities in your body. Everything in your body is connected and there are feedback mechanisms operating that relay messages backwards and forwards, so if you can change a number of factors at the same time, the effect could be really quite significant. It won't be long before you are able to completely stop the vicious PCOS circle your body has been stuck in, and start to create a positive upward spiral of health.

CHAPTER 5

HOW TO USE SUPPLEMENTS AND HERBS

My nutritional approach to tackling PCOS is specifically designed to make it as easy as possible for your body to rebalance itself. It is quite clear that diet can make an enormous difference to the symptoms of PCOS, your fertility and to your long-term health and risk of illness (see Chapter 4). But you really can boost the impact of these dietary changes by taking a special course of vitamins, minerals and herbs which support your body's natural functions and really help get your hormone levels back on track.

In theory, you should be able to get all the nutrients you need from your diet, but sadly, food today doesn't always contain good amounts of the key nutrients you need. Over-farming and the use of pesticides mean that much of the soil our food is grown in has become depleted in vital nutrients. Many fruits and vegetables at the supermarket have travelled great distances over many days to get to the shelves, with already meagre nutrients dwindling further still.

Our fruit and vegetables today contain an average of 20 per cent fewer minerals (magnesium 24 per cent, calcium 46 per cent, iron

27 per cent and zinc 59 per cent) than they did in the 1930s. Iron levels in modern meat are down by 47 per cent and in milk by over 60 per cent, while calcium levels in cheese in general are down by 15 per cent and Parmesan cheese by 70 per cent.[1] Many people are significantly deficient in certain vitamins and minerals (especially if they've dieted in the past), such as Omega 3 fats. This is particularly true if you have become what I call 'overfed and undernourished'. This happens if you eat more food than you need (causing weight gain). If the bulk of your diet is highly processed and refined, you may not be getting enough nutrients and you may end up overweight, and deficient in many key vitamins and minerals.

Many hormone systems in your body are dependent on certain nutrients in order to work properly; for instance, your reproductive hormones need zinc. So if you really do want to get your hormones back in balance and possibly also lose weight you will need to consider adding extra amounts of specific nutrients.

My recommendation, which is the same for all my PCOS patients, is to follow all the dietary suggestions in Chapter 4 *and* take a specific programme of supplements and herbs for three months. In my clinic, I test patients to assess specific deficiencies (I will discuss the most significant nutritional tests in Chapter 13), but you can make a big difference just by taking the key nutrients and herbs that we know to be important for PCOS.

Remember that supplements and herbs can never be a substitute for the dietary recommendations. They are, by definition, 'supplementary' to your food, but by working together with your new diet, there is no doubt in my mind that they will help balance your blood sugar, have a significant impact on your PCOS symptoms and improve your general health. Taken the right way, supplements and herbs can make your menstrual cycle more regular or kick-start a cycle if it has stopped. At the very least, you should notice some premenstrual changes such as breast tenderness, moodiness or vaginal mucus, which give you an indication that there has been a shift in your hormone levels.

Taking supplements is the best way to ensure you get the amounts of nutrients you need but if you also want to boost your intake through your meals I have included an easy-to-use list of food sources for different nutrients at the back of the book. See Appendix II on page 213.

If you are on the Pill, you will not notice any changes to your cycle, so I suggest you follow the dietary recommendations for three months and also add in the food supplements, but not the herbs (because of their possible hormone balancing effects). If you notice an improvement in your symptoms, you might want to come off the Pill, add in the herbs and give your body a chance to kick-start your periods.

SUPPLEMENTS

I always recommend that my patients buy the best-quality supplements they can afford because these are likely to contain high doses, in forms that are more easily absorbed by the body than cheap supplements. It really is worth making that investment if you want to turn your health around as quickly as possible.

Capsules are always better than tablets because your body doesn't have to work so hard to get at the nutrients (it merely has to melt the capsule, rather than try to break down a compressed tablet), and avoid chewable or fizzy tablets as they are usually packed with unwanted ingredients such as colourings and sugar or artificial sweeteners, which can exacerbate your problems rather than reduce them.

Here is my recommended supplement programme, including detailed information about each supplement and the required dosages.

YOUR PCOS SUPPLEMENT PROGRAMME AT A GLANCE

- **A good combination supplement** – containing chromium, the B vitamins B2, B3, B5, B6 and biotin, magnesium, zinc, manganese, co-enzyme Q10 and alpha-lipoic acid (as well as the herbs green tea extract and Siberian ginseng, see page 82).
- **Inositol (a B vitamin)**
- **Vitamin D**
- **Omega 3 fish oil**
- **Vitamin C**
- **Amino acid combination** – containing n-acetyl cysteine, arginine, carnitine, tyrosine, glutamine and the branched-chain amino acids, leucine, isoleucine and valine.
- **Probiotics**

BEST SUPPLEMENTS FOR PCOS

Chromium

I believe chromium is the key nutrient for PCOS as it helps to balance your blood sugar, improves insulin resistance, counteracts food cravings and is also useful for losing weight. It has been the most widely studied nutrient in blood-sugar control.[2] Chromium assists in the body's efficient use of insulin, which then controls your blood sugar. This mineral helps insulin move the sugar (glucose) from your blood into your cells.

It is quite common for us to be deficient in chromium because although the nutrient is found naturally in grains like rice and wheat, it is lost when those grains are refined – and we commonly consume refined grains.

Chromium is involved in your body's production of a substance called glucose tolerance factor (GTF) and this, in turn, aids the insulin your pancreas produces in being more effective. In this way, it helps reduce insulin resistance associated with PCOS, making your body more sensitive to insulin so that less needs to be produced and your blood-sugar levels are more balanced.[3]

If you have Type 2 diabetes, you may have low levels of chromium.[4] If you take chromium (combined with biotin – see below) it will improve your blood-sugar control.[5]

Take: 200µg of chromium daily.

Warning: if you are taking blood-sugar medication (such as metformin), speak to your doctor before taking a chromium supplement as its powerful effect may mean you need to adjust your dose of the drug.

B vitamins

The B vitamins in general are important in the reversal of PCOS symptoms. Vitamin B2 helps to turn fat, sugar and protein into energy, which makes it useful for both blood-sugar balance and weight control. B3 is a component of the glucose-tolerance factor (GTF – see page 70), which is released every time your blood sugar rises, and vitamin B3 is active in keeping the levels in balance. B3 is also useful in reducing LDL ('bad' cholesterol) and increasing HDL ('good' cholesterol).[6]

Vitamin B5 contributes to weight loss because it helps to control fat metabolism and plays a part in the healthy functioning of your adrenal glands. B6 is also needed for maintaining hormone balance and, together with B2 and B3, is essential for normal thyroid hormone production. Any deficiencies in these vitamins can affect thyroid function and, consequently, your metabolism and your weight. Vitamin B6, together with magnesium and zinc, contributes to the production of anti-inflammatory substances and reduces the amount of inflammation.

Make sure that you get your vitamin B12 levels checked if you are or have been on metformin (see page 34) as it is known that this drug increases the risk of a vitamin B12 deficiency.[7]

Biotin is also part of the B vitamin family, and when combined with chromium it is beneficial in balancing blood sugar and in carbohydrate metabolism. Biotin is also involved in the production of glucose and in assisting the body to use glucose effectively. Biotin is also valuable for reducing hair loss and for healthy nails.

Inositol is a B vitamin and a variation of it, called D-chiro-inositol, has been shown to help with PCOS by improving insulin sensitivity, regulating the cycle, inducing ovulation and reducing male hormones in both overweight and lean women with PCOS.[8] It is not possible to buy inositol in the form of D-chiro-inositol, but inositol seems to work just as well. Inositol taken by women with PCOS boosts weight loss and can improve ovulation frequency.[9]

Inositol is manufactured naturally in the body by the action of beneficial bacteria in the gut on the fibre in plants, and it is also found in healthy amounts in legumes and whole grains and in lecithin.
Take: 25mg of each of the B vitamins (B2, B3, B5 and B6) daily, 35μg of biotin, 200mg of inositol.

Vitamin D

Vitamin D, the 'sunshine' vitamin, is now recognized as being very active in controlling blood sugar and improving insulin sensitivity,[10] and research suggests that having good levels of vitamin D can help to prevent Type 2 diabetes.[11] Research has also shown that those with the highest levels of vitamin D are less likely to develop the condition.[12]

We also know that having low levels of vitamin D is associated with insulin resistance and obesity in women with PCOS.[13] And vitamin D is also involved in controlling the damaging inflammatory process throughout the body, increasing substances which are anti-inflammatory at the same time as reducing those that cause inflammation.

Vitamin D also plays a critical role in your body's ability to absorb calcium which is needed for healthy follicular development and maturation of the eggs in your ovaries. In one study, combining vitamin D with calcium resulted in normal menstrual cycles within two months for seven out of thirteen women, with two becoming pregnant.[14]

My recommendation is to do a simple home finger-prick test for vitamin D (see pages 192–3), so you know whether or not you are deficient. If your levels are low, I suggest adding in a separate vitamin D supplement for three months (on top of your multivitamin and mineral) and then retesting to make sure that the level is back to normal (for information on organizing the vitamin D test go to www.naturalhealthpractice.com).

Take: 400ius of vitamin D3 daily (or more if a blood test shows you to be deficient).

Magnesium

Magnesium is an important mineral for dealing with PCOS because it is involved in glucose metabolism. There is a strong link between magnesium levels and insulin resistance – the higher your magnesium levels the more sensitive you are likely to be to insulin.[15] Higher intakes of magnesium also help to reduce the risk of developing Type 2 diabetes, especially if you are overweight.[16]

Magnesium is crucial in its support of the adrenal glands, but stress can deplete natural levels of this mineral. It also plays a big role in producing anti-inflammatory prostaglandins, so has a part in controlling the damaging inflammation process.

Take: 40mg of magnesium daily (as magnesium citrate – see page 78).

Zinc

Zinc helps enormously with PCOS as it is instrumental in the production of your reproductive hormones; it also regulates your blood sugar by assisting insulin in its job and moving glucose (blood sugar) from your blood into your cells.

The mineral is also important for appetite control as a deficiency can cause a loss of taste and smell, creating a craving for stronger-tasting foods, including those that are saltier, fattier and more sugary. And it functions together with vitamins A and E in the manufacture of your thyroid hormones which control your metabolism and your weight. Zinc also helps to control appetite and hunger by affecting a hormone called leptin which is produced by fat cells and tells you when you have had enough to eat and feel satisfied; supplementing can increase leptin,[17] encouraging you not to overeat.

Finally, zinc plays a part in coping with stress and, together with magnesium and vitamin B6, it's involved in the body's production of anti-inflammatory substances.

Take: 15mg of zinc daily (as zinc citrate – see page 78).

Manganese

Manganese helps to balance your blood sugar and with healthy thyroid function and improves your body's ability to burn your food as energy.

Take: 5mg of manganese daily (as manganese citrate – see page 78).

Co-enzyme Q10

Co-enzyme Q10 is a substance that your body produces in nearly every cell. It breaks down carbohydrates and turns them into energy instead of being stored as fat. It also helps to balance your blood sugar,[18] lowering both glucose and insulin.

Take: 25mg of co-enzyme Q10 daily.

Alpha-lipoic acid

This powerful antioxidant contributes to regulating your blood-sugar levels because it releases energy by burning glucose, and it also helps to make you more insulin sensitive.[19] In addition, it has an effect on weight loss because if the glucose is being used for energy, your body releases less insulin and you then store less fat.

The other benefit of this antioxidant is that it supports your liver function, which means that this vital organ can more easily detoxify unwanted hormones.

Take: 100mg of alpha-lipoic acid daily.

Warning: if you are taking any medication that has an effect on your blood sugar (such as metformin), you need to speak to your doctor before supplementing with alpha-lipoic acid because it can lower blood-glucose levels, so you may need to be monitored and your medication possibly altered accordingly.

> To save you taking all of these nutrients separately, I have formulated a combination for the supplement company NHP called Nutri Support, available from your local health food shop or from www.naturalhealthpractice.com.

Omega 3 fats

These important fatty acids are absolutely crucial in the treatment of PCOS. They will help your body become more sensitive to insulin and play a strong role in controlling the destructive inflammatory process.

Omega 3 fats taken in supplement form have been found to reduce testosterone levels in women with PCOS and the greatest reduction is seen in those who previously had high levels of Omega 6 fats compared to Omega 3 (see page 194 for more information on the Omega 3 to 6 ratio).[20]

Take: 770mg EPA and 510mg DHA (see page 78) of fish oil daily. (I recommend NHP's Omega 3 Support, available from your local health food store or from www.naturalhealthpractice.com.) If you would like a vegetarian option then use 1,000mg of flaxseed (linseed) oil daily.

Vitamin C

Most animals produce vitamin C in their bodies by converting glucose to vitamin C but we humans have to get vitamin C from our food or supplements.

Many people take it to boost the immune system and prevent colds or flu but it is also useful for controlling PCOS by regulating glucose and insulin. Women with PCOS have lower levels of vitamin C than women without PCOS so this is a particularly important supplement for you.[21]

Incidentally, research has also shown that having good levels of vitamin C in the body can help to prevent diabetes,[22] and can help you burn more fat when you exercise, enabling you to lose weight faster.[23] **Take:** 500mg of vitamin C (as ascorbate rather than ascorbic acid) twice daily.

Amino acids

Amino acids are the building blocks of protein in your diet. Of the twenty-five amino acids, eight are classed as 'essential' because they can't be made naturally by your body. Certain amino acids can be very beneficial for PCOS as they can improve your insulin sensitivity and can also have an effect on weight loss (see Chapter 6).

N-acetyl cysteine

N-acetyl cysteine is a form of the amino acid cysteine which helps with the metabolism of the Omega 3 fats found in oily fish and linseed (flaxseed). It is also a powerful antioxidant and is active in reducing inflammation. In women with PCOS, N-acetyl cysteine aids in lowering insulin levels and makes the body more sensitive to it.[24]

This amino acid has also been used in women with PCOS who are resistant to clomiphene citrate (Clomid) and who have had a form of fertility surgery called ovarian drilling (see page 177). After the drilling procedure the women given N-acetyl cysteine (rather than a placebo) showed a significantly higher increase in both ovulation and pregnancy rates and lower incidence of miscarriage.[25]

Take: 500mg of N-acetyl cysteine daily.

Warning: if you are taking medication that affects your blood sugar (e.g. metformin), you should speak to your doctor before supplementing with N-acetyl cysteine.

Arginine

Arginine can be useful in reversing insulin resistance. It is involved in the release of glucagon (the opposite hormone to insulin), which helps your body burn fat stores. This also makes it useful for weight control. In addition, arginine helps your body build muscle (see Chapter 7), which is important for burning fat.

In one study, a combination of both arginine and N-acetyl cysteine was given to women with PCOS. The two amino acids helped to improve blood sugar and insulin control and also increased the number of menstrual cycles and ovulation, with one woman in a study of eight becoming pregnant on the second month.[26]

Take: 200mg of arginine daily.

Warning: arginine should not be used if you are susceptible to herpes as it can trigger the virus.

Carnitine

Carnitine assists the body's breakdown of fat to release energy and can also improve insulin sensitivity.

Take: 200mg of carnitine daily.

Tyrosine

Tyrosine is helpful for women with PCOS who are overweight as it is active in suppressing the appetite and burning off fat. It also plays a big role in the healthy functioning of the thyroid gland, so helps to improve metabolism.

Take: 200mg of tyrosine daily.

Glutamine

This amino acid is useful for helping with sugar cravings as it can be converted to sugar for energy and so takes away the need to eat something sweet. It also helps to build and maintain muscle which is key in fat burning.

Take: 200mg of glutamine daily.

TIPS FOR CHOOSING FOOD SUPPLEMENTS

- Avoid minerals in the form of oxides, sulphates and carbonates, which are difficult for your body to absorb. Choose those in the form of citrates instead. It is estimated that you will absorb only 6 per cent magnesium when the mineral is in the form of magnesium oxide compared to 90 per cent when it is magnesium citrate.
- Choose a natural form of vitamin E (labelled d-alpha-tocopherol) rather than the synthetic version (Dl-alpha-tocopherol), which is not so easily absorbed.
- Choose vitamin B6 as pyridoxal-5-phosphate, not the cheaper pyridoxine as it is easier for your body to use.
- Buy vitamin D as D3 (cholecalciferol), not the cheaper D2 (ergocalciferol) as D3 is 87 per cent more effective in raising and maintaining vitamin D levels than D2.[27]
- With vitamin C, choose a brand that offers it as ascorbate instead of ascorbic acid).
- When buying fish oils, check EPA and DHA levels on the label and aim for 770mg EPA and 510mg DHA per day. Avoid cod-liver oils, which are extracted from the liver of the fish (its waste disposal unit), rather than the body, because they can contain higher levels of toxins such as PCBs, dioxins and heavy metals such as mercury.
- Avoid probiotic drinks which can be loaded with sugar. Instead, choose a supplement that does not contain maltodextrin (it's high GI and can affect blood-sugar levels) but does contain FOS (fructooligosaccharides), which is classed as a prebiotic. This means that the beneficial bacteria (probiotics) use it as a 'food' to support their growth. Look for a brand that contains at least 22 billion organisms (including both lactobacillus and bifidobacteria strains) and does not have to be refrigerated because the contents are freeze dried, which makes it much more convenient especially when travelling.

Branched-chain amino acids (BCAAs)

BCAAs include three amino acids – leucine, isoleucine and valine. These are significant in PCOS because they help to balance blood sugar and good levels of them can have a beneficial effect on body weight.[28]
Take: 100mg of each of these three amino acids daily.

You do not have to take all these amino acids separately as there are many combination supplements available. The one I use in the clinic is NHP'S Amino Support, available from your local health food shop or from www.naturalhealthpractice.com.

Probiotics

Beneficial bacteria, also known as probiotics, play a part in reducing inflammation and can also help to control weight. We know that there is a difference between the composition of the gut flora in people of normal weight and those who are obese.[29] Poor levels of beneficial bacteria can make your body store more calories and can actually cause you to become overweight by increasing your appetite and making you more insulin resistant.[30]

We also know that probiotics can help to reduce weight around the middle of the body (more common in PCOS weight gain).[31]
Take: a probiotic that contains at least 22 billion organisms and does not have to be refrigerated – avoid the yogurt drinks that might contain sugar. I recommend NHP's Advanced Probiotic Support, available from health food shops or from www.naturalhealthpractice.com.

I use supplements from a number of different companies including NHP, BioCare and Solgar (available at www.naturalhealth-practice.com). I have also formulated some very high quality supplements exclusively for NHP containing the combinations and dosage levels I recommend (see Useful Resources, page 217).

HERBS

Herbs are extremely useful in the treatment of PCOS as they can directly target the hormone imbalances that cause many of the symptoms. They can be taken in tincture form (where they have been preserved with alcohol) or in capsules (vegetarian, preferably) filled with the dried herb. Again, I would suggest you avoid herbs that come in tablet form, as it is likely that other ingredients that may not be desirable will have been added and the tablets will also be more difficult to absorb.

As with supplements, I recommend you buy the best quality you can and organic where possible. Avoid brands with 'standardized extract' on the label. This means that the active ingredient in the herbal remedy is at a guaranteed dose, but you are not necessarily getting other parts of the herb (in natural proportions), which may play a big role in its function.

See below for my recommended herb programme, followed by detailed information about each herb and required dosages.

YOUR PCOS HERB PROGRAMME AT A GLANCE
- **A good combination supplement** – containing black cohosh, agnus castus and milk thistle
- **Saw palmetto** – taken separately as not every woman with PCOS will need this herb
- **Green tea** – taken separately or as part of your combination supplement (see page 82)
- **Siberian ginseng** – taken separately or as part of your combination supplement (see page 82)

THE BEST HERBS FOR PCOS
Black cohosh (Cimicifuga racemosa)
This herb is extremely important for PCOS as it helps to reduce the hormone LH which is often too high (see page 15). It is also beneficial for reducing anxiety and tension.

In 2006 there were concerns about black cohosh and liver disease. The National Institutes of Health in the US believes there's no case to answer; their website states that black cohosh has few side effects and that there is no scientific evidence to show that the herb causes liver damage (see www.nccam.nih.gov/health/blackcohosh for more details). In the UK, black cohosh is readily available but must carry an advisory warning stating that it 'may rarely cause liver problems'.

Take: 1 teaspoon of black cohosh as a tincture or 250–350mg in capsule form, twice daily.

Agnus castus (Vitex/chastetree berry)

This is the herb that helps to balance hormones and regulate the menstrual cycle because it works directly on the pituitary gland. The pituitary gland then sends message down to the ovaries, so if the right messages are getting to the ovaries they are more likely to function normally and healthily.

Take: 1 teaspoon of agnus castus as a tincture or 200–300mg in capsule form, twice daily.

Milk thistle (Silybum marianum)

This is one of the most crucial herbs for improving liver function. As the liver is the main organ of detoxification, this herb is extremely useful in the treatment of PCOS.

Take: 1 teaspoon of milk thistle as a tincture or 200–400mg in capsule form, twice daily.

Saw palmetto (Serenoa repens)

Saw palmetto can decrease the levels of 'male' hormones by working as an anti-androgen. It contributes to reducing levels of an enzyme which converts testosterone into its more active form that can target skin and hair follicles.

Take: 1 teaspoon of saw palmetto as a tincture or 200–300mg in capsule form, twice daily.

Warning: if you are taking medication that affects your hormones (the Pill or Mirena coil) then do not take the herbs mentioned above as their effects on hormones could clash.

Green tea extract

Green tea helps to control male hormones, inflammation and stress and can also aid weight loss. It contains an amino acid called L-theanine which has a relaxing effect on the body and mind. Green tea extract has also been shown to improve insulin sensitivity.[32]

Take: 50mg of green tea extract daily.

Siberian ginseng (Eleutherococcus senticosus)

This is the best herb for tackling stress, which can exacerbate PCOS symptoms. It is classed as an adaptogenic herb which means that it helps to create hormonal balance.

Note: women should avoid Panax ginseng (also called Asian, Chinese or Korean ginseng) as it appears to be much more suited to men.

Take: 100mg of Siberian ginseng daily.

Some of the herbs – like black cohosh and agnus castus – are more difficult to obtain because of recent EU legislation, but I am still able to use them in the clinic and they are available on certain good websites. The herbal combination I use in the clinic is NHP's Agnus Castus Support, which is a mix of five organic herbs, available from www.naturalhealthpractice.com. This same website also carries supplements and herbs from a number of excellent supplement companies (all of which I use in my clinics), so you can trust the quality of what you are buying.

I recommend that in conjunction with the seven dietary steps in Chapter 4, you take these recommended supplements and herbs for three months. I can almost guarantee you will feel a difference in your PCOS symptoms and a change in your body – the result of pure and natural dietary changes. If, however, you notice no improvement in your PCOS after six months I suggest you make an appointment to come into one of my clinics as you may need more individual guidance (for details, see page 217). Whatever the problem is, we will aim to help you.

OTHER NATURAL TREATMENTS

Other natural treatments such as acupuncture, homeopathy, osteopathy, aromatherapy, reflexology and hypnotherapy can be extremely helpful for PCOS and they can be used together with the nutritional and herbal recommendations above.

With homeopathy it is preferable to have an individual consultation with a practitioner, but remedies such as Sepia and Lachesis are often used for PCOS.

A review of the acupuncture studies on PCOS showed that it can be effective in improving blood flow to the ovaries and reducing their size, and with controlling blood sugar and insulin sensitivity.[33]

Aromatherapy oils, including fennel, clary sage and myrrh, can be helpful in balancing hormones. You can either add five drops of each to your bath or to 30ml of sweet almond oil and massage into your abdomen.

CHAPTER 6

CONTROLLING YOUR WEIGHT

Not every woman with PCOS will have a weight problem, but very often the two go hand in hand, so this chapter is specifically for you if you suffer with both.

Studies repeatedly show that losing weight is a really significant step towards improving the symptoms of PCOS.[1] Weight loss helps to decrease testosterone and insulin levels, increase levels of the beneficial protein SHBG and diminish excess hair and acne.[2]

If fertility is a problem, be comforted: studies show that losing just 5 per cent of your body weight can be enough to help stimulate ovulation, give you regular cycles, reduce the number of micro follicles on the ovaries and help you to conceive.[3] In one study, 82 per cent of the women started to ovulate after losing weight,[4] and 90 per cent, who had previously not been ovulating, conceived naturally.[5]

Having set the scene, I must also say that you should not be too hard on yourself about your weight. When you have PCOS, weight gain is much harder to avoid, and much, much harder to shift than it is for other women. Research has shown that a woman with PCOS can eat the same amount of calories as a woman without PCOS, but still gain more weight.[6]

It doesn't seem fair and, in my opinion, it certainly isn't. Yours is a metabolic problem. Your hormones are out of balance. But you don't have to go on a rigid calorie-counting diet. Trust me, when you address that hormonal imbalance, your weight will automatically drop.

It is extremely important for any weight loss to be gradual. You could crash diet and lose pounds very quickly, but they rarely stay off and, particularly if you have PCOS, you could quite easily end up with more weight gain than you had in the first place.[7] If you allow yourself to feel hungry, your body thinks it is experiencing a famine, which puts it under undue stress and raises those erratic hormones even more.

LOSING BODY FAT

Everyone talks about trying to lose weight, but your focus should be specifically on losing body fat. The usual way of assessing whether you are overweight is to calculate your Body Mass Index (BMI), which is the ratio of your height to weight (see box).

CALCULATING BMI

To calculate your BMI you need to divide your weight in kg by the square of your height in metres. So if your weight is 63.5kg (10 stone) and your height is 1.68m (5ft 6in), your BMI is $63.5 \div (1.68 \times 1.68) = 22.5$.

BMI is split into five categories:
- Under 20: underweight
- 20–25: normal
- 25–30: overweight
- 30–40: obese
- Over 40: dangerously obese

But BMI is a poor measure. It cannot distinguish between muscle and fat. Muscle is heavier than fat, so the more muscle you have, the heavier you will be. This means that a very fit athlete packed with muscle may have the same BMI as a couch potato with a lot of body fat.

Muscle is important because it is metabolically active – it actually burns calories even when you are doing nothing. So the more muscle you have, the more body fat you burn.

And your body is really clever: if you are on a crash diet, it will sense that you are losing weight quickly, but does not know that you are doing this deliberately. Being programmed for survival, your body's main aim is to keep you alive, so when it senses that you have lost over 10 per cent of your body weight, it will slow down your metabolism by as much as 15 per cent to reduce the amount of energy you are using, so that you can survive while there is a 'shortage' of food.

Once you've crash dieted, when you start eating normally again, the weight you have lost will very usually go straight back on as fat. Your body thinks food is plentiful again, so it must restock the fat stores because it does not know when the next 'famine' could be.

It is not physically possible to lose more than 2lb (1kg) *of fat* a week. Any more than that and you will be losing muscle and water. So aim to lose fat gradually, so the body doesn't register famine. That way you will get slim and stay slim – permanently.

DON'T WEIGH YOURSELF

I don't recommend that you weigh yourself. Instead, get some scales that measure your body-fat percentage (Tanita is a good make to try) or use a tape measure.

The fat-measuring scales work by sending an electric current (painlessly!) up one leg and down the other. Because muscle is a better conductor of electricity than fat, the more fat you have the longer it takes for the current to pass through one leg back to the other. Women aged between eighteen and thirty-nine should aim for a body-fat percentage of between 21 and 32 per cent, while between age forty and fifty-nine the healthy range is 23–33 per cent.

Alternatively, because PCOS leaves women with a tendency for fat to accumulate around the middle, you could just use a tape measure. Simply measure your waist and then your hips and divide your hip measurement into your waist measurement. So if you have a 34in (86cm) waist and 37in (94cm) hips your waist-to-hip ratio is 0.9. A healthy ratio is less than 0.8.

Either weigh yourself using fat-measuring scales or use your tape measure regularly to monitor how much fat you are losing.

PCOS AND WEIGHT GAIN

There are a number of theories as to why PCOS makes you more sensitive to weight gain regardless of the amount of food you eat.

1. THRIFTY GENES
In some cultures where food is often scarce, people develop a certain genetic make-up which allows them to survive famines. Their metabolism becomes extremely efficient at converting food into fat, so their bodies have a store for when food is in short supply. These people have what is called 'thrifty genes'. But when food is abundant the people with thrifty genes put on weight quickly and end up with a higher risk of Type 2 diabetes.

Many experts think PCOS could be linked to this thrifty gene, and it certainly helps to explain why PCOS is more common on certain continents, such as Asia, for example.

Some believe PCOS is linked to 'fertility-first genes'.[8] The theory suggests that having this specific cluster of genes enables women to conserve energy for reproduction when food is scarce, so putting them at an advantage for survival. But having these 'fertility-first genes' becomes a disadvantage in modern societies where food is abundant. It also twists the logic in women with PCOS because the more weight they gain, the more their fertility seems to suffer.

2. SLUGGISH METABOLISM

Weight gain is linked to metabolism, and metabolism is linked to the action of the thyroid gland. So if you have PCOS, you should get your thyroid function checked. It may be worth asking your GP to check for thyroid antibodies, as well as the thyroid hormone levels. Women with PCOS have a higher risk of suffering from autoimmune thyroid disease,[9] which means that your own cells attack your thyroid. Some studies suggest that if you don't have enough progesterone (common in PCOS because you don't produce this hormone), you could be more susceptible to this autoimmune problem. Healthy thyroid function is essential for ovulation and fertility.

Get your vitamin D level checked too because a deficiency in this nutrient has been linked to autoimmune conditions. (A simple vitamin D home finger-prick test is available from www.naturalhealth practice.com.)

3. HUGE APPETITE

Your appetite is controlled by the hypothalamus in the brain, but there are a number of other factors at play as well.

There are many chemical messengers and hormones that control your appetite. They are vital for survival because they tell you when you are hungry and also when you are satisfied and should stop eating. The two most important ones are ghrelin, which makes you hungry and leptin, which makes you feel satisfied.

Ghrelin

Ghrelin is produced in your stomach. It makes you feel hungry and starts the secretion of gastric juices ready to digest the food you are about to eat. Levels are typically higher just before eating and then drop off afterwards. However, if you have PCOS, your ghrelin levels are less likely to drop, so you could feel permanently hungry.[10]

Leptin

Leptin is a hormone produced by your fat cells that helps to control your appetite and your weight. The more fat you have the more leptin you produce.

You'd think this would put you at an advantage, but leptin is a bit like insulin – if you have too much you can become leptin resistant. This means that leptin does not send the right messages to your brain and you never feel satisfied with what you have eaten. We know that overweight women with PCOS tend to have higher leptin levels than normal-weight women with PCOS.[11] Also, the inflammatory process triggered by PCOS can make you more leptin resistant, causing you to eat more, gain weight and leave you stuck in a vicious cycle, so make sure you follow all the recommendations on page 64 for controlling inflammation. And it really is a good idea to get your vitamin D levels checked (see pages 192–3) because low levels of vitamin D in PCOS are connected to being overweight and higher leptin levels.[12]

WEIGHT-LOSS TIPS

Try these simple tips to help control your appetite, reduce cravings and binges and make weight-loss easier.

WHAT TO EAT

Here are some practical ways you can use certain foods and drinks in order to help with weight loss.

Soup

If you have soup before a meal, you should end up eating fewer calories during the meal because soup stops the cells in the stomach producing your hunger hormone ghrelin and turns off your appetite.

Studies show that the body registers greater satisfaction when food is liquidized, and soup moves out of the stomach more gradually than a solid meal would, leaving you feeling more satisfied for longer.

Porridge

The University of Sydney put together a chart of foods that make us feel more satisfied and in it porridge was listed as twice as filling as muesli, due to its consistency. Avoid the instant type of porridge, which breaks the oats down into finer particles and also pre-cooks them, so they lack the slow-release quality of regular oats. They also often have added salt and sweeteners.

Green tea

Green tea has a fat-burning effect which could support weight loss. It can also help reduce levels of LDL ('bad' cholesterol).[13]

Cinnamon

Cinnamon has been shown to improve insulin sensitivity and has a fat-burning effect (see page 51).[14]

Sweet potato

Unlike ordinary potatoes, sweet potatoes are low GI, and they trigger the release of a hormone called adiponectin which helps to regulate insulin and improve insulin sensitivity.[15]

Grapefruit

Grapefruit may be useful for weight loss and also insulin resistance. It contains high concentrations of a flavonoid called naringenin which may act on liver cells and prevent rises in glucose. One study showed that three grapefruit halves or a glass of the juice at each meal improved weight loss as compared with not including grapefruit (the best results were with the fresh fruit rather than juice).[16]

Warning: grapefruit juice can interfere with the breakdown of certain drugs like aspirin and the Pill, leaving you with higher concentrations in your blood.[17]

Vinegar and lemon juice

Adding vinegar or lemon juice to your food can lower the glycaemic index (GI) of that food by 20 to 40 per cent.[18] Vinegar is also thought to slow down the rate at which food leaves your stomach.[19]

Coconut oil

Coconut oil does contain saturated fat, but nearly half of the fatty acids in coconut are lauric acid which can be easily converted into energy by the body. It is thought to promote thermogenesis, which increases metabolism and produces energy, and is also particularly good for cooking as, unlike many other oils, it doesn't produce harmful free radicals when heated to a high temperature.

Fibre

Fibre that naturally occurs within food can give you a sense of fullness and so help to control your appetite and hunger. (I don't recommend bran on its own, however, as it can irritate the digestive tract, causing bloating and flatulence.) A study of over 110,000 people showed that those who included whole grains in their diet had lower BMI and less fat around the middle.[20]

Protein with every meal

Protein slows the rate of digestion, lowering the GI of any meal, keeping blood sugar in balance and reducing the need for so much insulin to be produced.

Protein (in the form of fish, eggs, or nuts, seeds, beans and quinoa) also makes you feel more satisfied and will leave you feeling fuller for longer, so helping to control your appetite and stop you overeating. This is particularly useful if you have PCOS,[21] and it also addresses symptoms that might normally sabotage a diet, such as cravings.[22]

Almonds are a great source of protein and they also appear to improve insulin sensitivity,[23] as well as helping to reduce blood glucose levels and make you feel more satisfied when added to a meal. And, contrary to what you might think, they can aid in weight loss. A study showed that eating twenty-three almonds per day not only contributes to reducing body-fat percentage, but also lowers cholesterol, LDL ('bad') cholesterol and insulin.[24] Twenty-three a day is the suggested optimum amount, and if they are consumed as snacks, they will give you more control over your appetite by making you feel more full and less hungry.

Studies also show that almonds and walnuts can increase levels of SHBG and reduce levels of androgens in women with PCOS.[25]

Resistant starch

The GI of any carbohydrate depends on the type of starch it contains. But not all starch is rapidly converted to glucose. In fact, a significant proportion of certain dietary starches escapes digestion and absorption in your small intestines and reaches your large intestines essentially intact. This kind of starch is called resistant starch because it is resistant to your stomach acid and digestive enzymes and survives right through the digestive tract without being broken down.

Resistant starch behaves in a similar way to fibre, making you feel fuller and keeping your bowels moving regularly and comfortably. This kind of starch is important if you have PCOS as it helps to prevent weight gain. The World Health Organization has even stated that it is the only dietary constituent which shows a convincing protective effect against weight gain.[26] Resistant starch also appears to aid in controlling your blood sugar[27] and helps to improve insulin sensitivity.[28]

There are two forms of starch: amylose and amylopectin. Amylose is the most resistant because it is a tighter molecule and harder for your body to break down. Most starchy carbohydrates will contain a mixture of both amylose and amylopectin, so it is useful to choose those with more amylose such as beans, peas, oats and green bananas.

Unfortunately, wheat is high in amylopectin, which means it can be converted to glucose much faster than rice and oats. Wholewheat is definitely better, but I recommend PCOS sufferers avoid wheat to achieve the fastest possible weight loss.

When potatoes are cooked and then left to cool the starch that is formed by the cooling process becomes resistant to digestion. So if you want to eat potatoes it's far better to eat them cold in a potato salad (with protein, of course). The same goes for white rice or pasta; so if you have a craving you really can't ignore, opt for sushi or a cold pasta salad.

Supplements and Herbs

There are many supplements and herbs that will help your weight loss. See Chapter 5.

STOP BEATING YOURSELF UP

Don't be too hard on yourself: you aren't 'bad' if you indulge now and again and you are not 'good' if you stick to vegetables and fruit for every meal. Ditch the guilt!

I recommend an 80/20 rule: as long as you eat healthily 80 per cent of the time, you can afford the odd indulgence. And when you do indulge, make sure you choose the best-quality treat you can afford and savour every mouthful!

WHAT *NOT* TO EAT

There are certain foods and patterns of eating that can make it harder to lose weight and I have covered the most important ones below.

Artificial sweeteners

These increase your appetite and make you eat more (see pages 46–7 for more information).

Fruit juice

A gulp of fruit juice will hike your blood sugar levels fairly quickly (albeit less than ordinary sugar), and too much juice each day can cause resistance to the appetite-suppressing hormone leptin. Even though fructose is a fruit sugar, it is no better for someone with PCOS than any other form of sugar.

Fruit juice may not cause blood glucose to rise as quickly as ordinary sugar, but your body moves it straight to your liver where it forms fats and can increase the liver's production of cholesterol. It can also exacerbate insulin resistance by triggering the release of both cortisol (the stress hormone) and insulin.

Carbohydrates after 6pm

The body finds it easier to digest food and burn off calories during the day when you are active, so it is a good idea to avoid eating after 8pm (apart from a small snack before bed if you typically wake up in the night). Starchy carbohydrates (pasta, potatoes, bread) eaten late in the day will hike insulin levels and increase the chance of fat storage. So I recommend avoiding unrefined carbohydrates after 6pm for the first four weeks of this regime to allow your body to work as efficiently as possible.

HOW TO EAT

It's not just what you eat but also how you eat that can make a difference to losing weight quickly. Bear in mind the following points whenever you eat.

Eat slowly and chew well

The chemical cholecystokinin (CCK) is released as food enters the stomach. It tells your digestion to slow down and subsequently gives the message to your brain that you are full, allowing your appetite to naturally decrease. This message takes about twenty minutes, so if you eat quickly you could end up eating far more than you need to before your body gets around to telling you to stop. You should also leave time at the end of a meal for your body to register that you are full before you reach for that rich dessert.

Sit down when you eat and take your time. Eating on the run is not good for general health and appetite control.

Use smaller plates

Research shows that the larger our plates, the more food we put on them, and the more we eat – regardless of appetite![29]

Little and often

If you can convince your body that there's no shortage of food, it won't have to hold on to fat stores, and will boost your metabolism so it uses the food you do eat as energy instead of storing it as fat.

Have a healthy breakfast followed by a mid-morning snack, lunch, a mid-afternoon snack and supper. Don't leave more than three hours between meals and snacks.

This pattern of eating ensures that insulin levels stay low after a meal and more calories are burned.[30]

Keep a food diary

I ask all my patients to record exactly what they've eaten in the days leading up to their appointment with me and they usually tell me they are quite shocked when they see their typical diet in writing.

This can be enough to make you think about what you're doing and to stop you making unhealthy food choices.

Photograph your plate

Studies show that taking a photograph of everything you eat, just before you eat it, concentrates the mind to eat healthier foods, and can put paid to a potential bingeing spree.[31]

HOW *NOT* TO EAT

There are certain types of behaviour that you should avoid when aiming to lose weight. They might simply be bad habits that have built up over the years but they can often sabotage your good efforts, so try to change them if you can.

Mindlessly

Studies show we eat up to 70 per cent more than we realize if distracted by the TV, while eating lunch in front of your computer makes you less likely to remember what you have eaten and more likely to feel hungry later. In one study computer users ate twice as many biscuits half an hour after lunch at their desk than the non-computer users.[32]

For comfort

When you do get a craving, stop and think, are you really hungry or are you feeling lonely, scared, guilty or angry? Recognizing the difference is half the battle. If you do eat when you feel lonely or angry, try to think of other ways to change that feeling – perhaps a quick walk, dancing to music or phoning a friend.

When stressed

The stress hormone cortisol blocks the action of leptin (which you need to reduce appetite and body fat) if your body thinks you really need to refuel after a stressful event. This reaction isn't helpful if your stress involved worrying rather than physically fighting for your life, and can make it much more likely that you will gain weight.

Try to get a little 'me time', and make sure you are taking stress-busting magnesium and B vitamins in your supplement mix. Use the suggestions in Chapter 9 to control your stress levels as best you can.

Skipping breakfast

Many patients tell me they simply aren't hungry first thing in the morning, and if they eat breakfast, they're likely to want to eat all day. But skipping breakfast is the worst thing you can do if you want to lose weight. It seriously increases the chance that you will be hungry mid-morning and reach for a high-sugar quick fix that sets you up for a blood-sugar rollercoaster all day. Research shows that dieters who eat breakfast are more successful than those who don't – and the more substantial the breakfast the better.

Missing meals

If you miss meals your body will think there is a shortage of food, will slow down your metabolism and hold on tight to your fat stores. Nothing is more likely than this to set up some serious cravings as your body desperately tries to correct the blood-sugar dips.

Counting calories

Not all calories are equal, and those from carbohydrates, protein or fats will have a different effect on your metabolism and your weight. A piece of fruit containing 100 calories, for example, will have a totally different impact on your body from a piece of cake (white flour and sugar) with the same calorie count. Research shows that overweight people on unlimited quantities of low-GI food lose more weight than overweight people on a low-fat, low-calorie diet.[33]

GET ENOUGH SLEEP

If you are not getting enough sleep, your body will produce more of the hunger hormone (ghrelin) and less leptin (which makes you feel full), so lack of sleep makes it much harder to lose weight. One study showed that people on a diet who slept for eight and a half hours lost 55 per cent more body fat than those who slept for just five and a half.[34] Not only does sleep deprivation make it harder for your body to let go of fat, it also makes you hungrier the next day, triggering cravings for sweets and refined white carbohydrates as you search for something to give yourself a quick lift.

Just one night of four hours of sleep is enough to start the insulin resistance process,[35] and if the lack of sleep continues over six nights, this sleep debt can reduce your ability to respond to insulin by 30 per cent.[36]

Practical tips for improving your sleep
1. Avoid any food or drink containing caffeine (tea, coffee, cola and chocolate) as the caffeine acts as a stimulant. Everybody's sensitivity to caffeine is different, but for some women a cup of coffee in the morning can be enough to prevent them from getting to sleep at night.
2. Eat little and often during the day to keep blood sugar steady, and prevent the adrenal glands from overworking. This should ensure that the hormone cortisol, which is produced from the adrenals, starts to wind down when you go to bed, as it should.
3. If you tend to wake in the middle of the night – especially if you wake abruptly and with palpitations – you could have nocturnal hypoglycaemia. Try having a small snack of complex carbohydrates, such as an oat cake or half a slice of

wheat or rye bread, about an hour before bed. This will stop your blood-sugar levels dropping overnight, and prevent adrenaline from being released into the bloodstream in an effort to correct this imbalance.

4. Avoid alcohol. Not only does it affect blood-sugar levels, which causes adrenaline to be released, but it also blocks the transport of tryptophan into the brain. Tryptophan is important because it is converted into serotonin, the calming and relaxing neurotransmitter.

5. Drink a cup of chamomile tea before bed to encourage relaxation.

6. Try to exercise early in the day. Some women may find it difficult to sleep following a late exercise session and vigorous activity can delay the secretion of melatonin which governs the body clock. By exercising in the morning, you will reinforce healthy sleeping habits that lead to regular melatonin production.[37]

7. A few drops of the aromatherapy oils bergamot, lavender, roman chamomile and marjoram in a warm bath, just before bed can encourage relaxation; or a few drops on your pillow at bedtime, or used in a vaporizer, can have the same effect. A pre-bed, gentle massage with the same oils will help to promote sleep.

8. Keep to a sleep routine, if possible setting your alarm for the same time each morning. Many women fall into a poor pattern, where they wake too early and then struggle to stay awake in the evenings. Sometimes it's useful to reprogramme your body clock, so you get the restful sleep when you want to – that is at night!

9. At least an hour before bed, write yourself a 'to-do' list, so that you avoid lying in bed mulling over what needs to be done as you go to sleep.

10. Sex or masturbation can help you go to sleep by relaxing you and releasing tension.

11. Herbs can be extremely effective for sleep-related problems. Hops, valerian, passionflower and skullcap all work as gentle sedatives, and can be of use in overcoming insomnia. Try not to rely on only one herb, but rotate among several, to ensure that you don't become overly dependent. Chamomile is another useful sedative, and it helps to calm and tone the nervous system, promoting restful sleep.

12. Magnesium, known as 'nature's tranquillizer', is good for sleep problems. If you suffer from restless legs or cramps, take both magnesium and vitamin E.

13. Learn to practise relaxation. Try lying on your back and, starting from your toes, work up your body, tensing each part and then relaxing it in turn, ending with your face. This enables you to feel the difference between tension and relaxation.

14. Use visualization techniques. Imagine yourself on a beautiful beach with the warm sun on your skin, soft sand under your feet, blue sky, clear water and the fragrant scent of wonderful coloured flowers. You could also have some soothing music playing while you let yourself go and imagine yourself in this tropical paradise. This technique is very useful if you have an active mind that simply won't switch off, even when you are physically tired. By focusing the mind on something relaxing, it becomes much easier for it to 'let go'.

15. Avoid watching TV or checking your mobile phone or computer from about an hour before you go to bed, so that you are not exposed to bright lights. Light exposure before bed can suppress the release of the hormone melatonin which helps you go to sleep.

SLIMMING DRUGS

There are drugs available to aid in losing weight, but I prefer my patients to stick to a healthy diet so they are better able to maintain the weight loss in the long term. All drugs carry side effects and you do have to come off them at some point, so it's far better to get into good eating habits for life.

Orlistat

This drug works by blocking the absorption of fat in the intestines. It has been used for weight loss in women with PCOS,[38] but if you don't stick to a low-fat diet you can suffer from diarrhoea, and other quite unpleasant side effects include anal leakage, flatulence and bowel pain. The other problem is that because Orlistat blocks the absorption of fat, the drug also blocks the absorption of the fat-soluble vitamins A, D and E which are crucial for your health.

Sibutramine

This appetite suppressant has been used in the treatment of obesity in women with PCOS,[39] but was withdrawn from the market in 2010 because of the increased risk of stroke and heart problems.

Metformin

Insulin is the 'fat storing' hormone and metformin is an insulin sensitiser, however, research shows that it does not necessarily help with weight loss.[40] If you are considering the use of drugs to help you lose weight, don't rely on metformin.

Note: for all these drugs, the PCOS consensus paper makes it clear that they should not be considered as first-line therapy for obesity in women with PCOS.[41] In some cases, drugs can be useful, but these should not be considered your only course of action for weight loss.

BARIATRIC SURGERY

Gastric band (bariatric) surgery, whereby various surgical techniques are used to reduce the size of the stomach by as much as 90 per cent, can be successful for women with PCOS who are morbidly obese.[42] When the stomach is made so much smaller, you can only eat tiny amounts of food before the stomach is stretched, stimulating nerves which send a message to the brain that the stomach is full.

But despite all the publicity surrounding celebrities who have had the procedure, bariatric surgery is a big step to take and should only be used as a last resort. There are risks inherent in any surgery, but in these procedures complications can be numerous. Also, the restricted diet can result in deficiencies in vitamin D, calcium, vitamin B12, folic acid and iron, so you may be put on food supplements for life.

CHAPTER 7

EXERCISE

When it comes to controlling your PCOS, the single most important lifestyle change you can make – after sorting out your diet, that is – is to exercise regularly. There's absolutely no doubt that exercise is vital for your health: it keeps your immune system functioning well, releases endorphins (the 'feelgood' brain chemicals), helps your bowels function efficiently and it's good for your bones and your heart. But we now also know that it provides an essential key to balancing the hormonal upheaval of PCOS.

Exercise – when combined with good dietary choices – can not only reverse the insulin resistance that blights PCOS sufferers, it can make their cells more sensitive to insulin. Added to which, it plays a crucial role in weight loss and really can boost fragile self-esteem.

And if, as a result of your PCOS, you are struggling to conceive, exercise can boost your chances of getting pregnant too.[1] This is particularly true if you, like many PCOS sufferers, appear to be resistant to the fertility drug clomiphene, which is often given to women in an attempt to stimulate the ovaries to produce more eggs (see page 174 for more information). Studies show that after six weeks of combining clomiphene with diet and exercise, overweight and obese women with PCOS stopped being resistant to the drug and significantly increased the chances that they would ovulate taking it.[2] So combining exercise, diet and supplements gives you the best possible chance of conceiving naturally.

Be warned, however, that some forms of exercise work better than others. I see many women in the clinic who spend an hour in the gym up to three times a week and feel they are doing a vigorous workout, but still can't shift their excess weight – particularly that around the middle of the body. It is very common for women with PCOS to become 'apple shaped' with fat gathering on their tummy, hips, chest and back. This is caused by the action of male hormones, and is particularly difficult to shift.

In this chapter I will show why exercise is vital if you have PCOS (whether you are overweight or not) and how to do the right kind of exercise for weight loss. This is particularly important if you are time poor. You need to know you are using your time efficiently, and that whatever time you do spend exercising is absolutely worthwhile.

So the best approach is to use the dietary recommendations from Chapter 4, follow the supplement programme (Chapter 5) and exercise not only to improve your PCOS symptoms, but also to help with weight loss.[3]

Some exercises, like yoga and t'ai chi, are good for you whether you need to lose weight or not. They can induce relaxation because they involve slow, controlled movements with deep breathing. Relieving stress can also lead to reduced inflammation, which is useful if you have PCOS.[4] Other exercises, such as Pilates and using large stability balls, can improve your core strength (strengthening the muscles around the middle of the body) and are worth considering too.

But don't be fooled into thinking you can lose fat around your middle by doing stomach crunches alone. The trick is to lose the belly fat first (by following the dietary recommendations and exercises in this book), then add stomach crunches to tone your abdominal muscles.

EXERCISE IF YOU DON'T NEED TO LOSE WEIGHT

With PCOS, even if you are not overweight, you can still be insulin resistant, so your exercise programme should aim to make your body become more insulin sensitive, as well as keeping you in good health (and preventing weight gain which would worsen your PCOS symptoms).

If weight is not an issue for you, your emphasis should be very much on aerobic exercise such as walking, jogging, cycling, dancing, swimming or an active exercise class. Regularly exercising like this will increase the number of glucose transporters in your muscles, making them more receptive to insulin. This means that your pancreas should not have to produce as much insulin to get the same response. The exercise will reduce both your blood sugar and insulin.

I suggest you aim for at least thirty minutes of fast-paced activity every day.

EXERCISE IF YOU DO NEED TO LOSE WEIGHT

The key to using exercise to help you lose weight (fat) is to build muscle. Muscle is metabolically active, so the more muscle you have, the more calories you will burn (even when you're not exercising): 450g (1lb) of muscle burns 75 calories a day compared to the same weight of fat, which burns 8 calories a day.

Muscle also takes up five times less space than fat, so if you lose fat, but gain muscle, you should see inch losses especially around the middle of your body. But muscle weighs more than fat, so if you weigh yourself instead of using either the body-fat percentage or waist-to-hip ratio (see pages 87–8) you may think exercise is not working for you – but it is!

Aerobic exercise is not great for building muscle and if you are trying to lose weight through aerobic (cardiovascular) exercise, you'll need to spend a large part of your day doing it. The rule is that your body only starts to plunder your fat reserves once you have been exercising for 20 minutes, and even if you exercise vigorously you will only then be using up very few calories. Thirty minutes jogging on a treadmill burns about 200 calories – equivalent to two cappuccinos (without added sugar) or two glasses of wine or half a muffin. So if you typically grab a coffee and a cake after each gym session, you can easily put on more than you have burned off. To burn one pound of body fat (which is about 3,555 calories) you'd need to do about eighteen thirty-minute aerobic sessions.

To use exercise effectively to lose weight, you need to do two things:

1. Regular aerobic (cardiovascular) exercise, with interval training.
2. Regular anaerobic exercise to build muscle, with resistance training.

All the research suggests that a combination of both aerobic and anaerobic exercise gives the best loss, in both fat and inch terms, and has the most beneficial effect on blood-sugar levels.[5]

AEROBIC (CARDIOVASCULAR) EXERCISE WITH INTERVAL TRAINING

Interval training is defined as varying the intensity of an exercise programme so that you work at maximum effort for thirty to sixty seconds, then drop back to a more comfortable level to catch your breath, before pushing yourself hard for a set amount of time again. This effectively 'shakes' your body out of its exercise habits. Experts call this 'metabolic disturbance'. If you do the same set of exercises at the gym, or the same class every time, your body will swiftly adapt, and arrange itself so it uses the minimum possible energy to complete the task asked of it. It's a very clever survival mechanism, designed to avoid wasting precious resources. If you jump on the treadmill every time you go to the gym and run for thirty minutes at the same speed, your body will become incredibly efficient, use up less energy and burn fewer calories which means less weight loss. But turning up the dial so you sprint occasionally will really shake things up, improve your fitness, and ensure that you burn calories (albeit to a lesser extent) for up to twenty-four hours *after* you stop exercising.

There are a number of different interval patterns you can use (on a treadmill, bike, swimming pool or just out jogging), but they usually involve a steady warm-up of about five minutes, followed by six to eight repetitions of very high-intensity exercise, interspersed with lower-intensity exercise and then a cool-down.

One of the most popular high-intensity trainings is Tabata, created by a Dr Izumi Tabata from Japan. The training only lasts for four minutes, but it can produce remarkable results. The Tabata training involves the following:

- Five minutes of warm-up.
- High-intensity for twenty seconds.
- Rest for ten seconds.
- Repeat this eight times (takes four minutes in total).
- Two minutes cool-down.

This type of interval training has been shown to be more effective at shifting weight (body fat) than long aerobic workouts.[6] One study showed that the body burns more fat when the intensity is higher and that weight loss continues after the exercise has finished; so that those four minutes of interval training are more effective than one hour of steady aerobic exercise.[7] It really does sound too good to be true, especially when government guidelines recommend thirty to sixty minutes of exercise every single day.

So how can a much shorter exercise programme be more effective than a longer one? The answer is because high-intensity interval training challenges your body to do something different every few seconds, so it can't get into a habit or adapt to the exercise and reduce the amount of energy it uses.

This doesn't diminish the health benefits of long walks (great for your general health, especially when in the open air), but if you want to lose weight with exercise you clearly have to do something different.

The other good thing about interval training is that it works for any kind of exercise in which you can vary the intensity. Use an exercise bike, a cross-trainer or a rowing machine, and aim for three of these short sessions a week.

If you haven't exercised for a while, you should ease into this gradually and not go at full pelt for the first few times. Try thirty seconds at moderate intensity, then rest for ninety seconds and repeat this three to eight times, until you feel you are ready to shorten the rest period.

Alternatively, try this treadmill workout:

- Start walking at 6kph or a level with which you are comfortable.
- After one minute change the speed to 6.5.
- After the next minute change to 7.0.
- After the next minute change to 7.5.
- After the next minute change to 8.0.
- After the next minute change to 8.5.
- After the next minute (so you have done five minutes in total), go back to 6kph.
- After the next minute repeat the cycle, changing to 6.5 and so on.

You should aim to keep this up for twenty to thirty minutes. And as you get fitter, you could start at 6.5kph, moving up each minute by 0.5 as before, then start at 7.0 or higher. This will keep your body 'on its toes', prevent you from getting too used to the workout and maintain your fat-burning mode. It also prevents you from getting too bored and makes a simple walk on the treadmill a bit more of a challenge. You can also vary the speeds and gaps as you get fitter to make it more challenging.

You can do interval training on an exercise bike at home or walking/jogging around a park, but I do think it is worth considering joining your local gym. Look out for 'pay-as-you-go' schemes at council-run gyms, as they represent good value and don't hook you into a year's membership. You will find people of all ages and sizes at the gym, so don't be afraid of standing out and do look into it.

ANAEROBIC EXERCISE WITH RESISTANCE TRAINING

Anaerobic exercise helps to build muscles by using free weights such as dumb bells or weight machines in the gym, or your own body weight (press-ups or lunges).

The more muscle you have, the faster your metabolism will be and the more fat you will burn. So even when you are not exercising, your muscles will be helping to keep your weight down. This is a great weapon in the battle against PCOS weight gain.

Try to find time for two to three thirty-minute sessions of weight training a week. Weight training actually tears the muscle fibres, which build up as they repair while you are resting, so it's best to avoid training the same muscle groups every day. Instead, vary the exercise groups and give your muscles the chance to recover and repair afterwards. Focus on your upper body in one session and lower body the next, so each muscle group has time to recover.

When using weights for the first time, always start with a light weight and build up slowly. The aim is to lift the weight twelve times (this is called a repetition or 'rep') and do three lots of these (called sets), with one minute's rest between sets. You'll know you have the right weight (for now) if you can only get to eight or ten reps in the third set. If you can do more than twelve reps in the third set, the weight is too light. You will quickly gain strength, however, so as soon as the third set becomes easier, increase the weight size or resistance.

If you join a gym, you will be given guidance on how to use the weights and the machines. Don't hesitate to ask if you are unsure because if your technique is not correct, you are unlikely to be getting the full benefit from your exercise and you could injure yourself.

EXERCISE TIPS

- Try and exercise on an empty stomach. The best time is before breakfast because you will burn more fat and it will help you to become more insulin sensitive.[8] If you are doing your aerobic and weight training exercises in the same session, always do the weight training first. Do a five-minute aerobic warm up, then go straight into the weight training. This ensures you aren't too tired to do the weight training properly, and in the aerobic session you will be burning more fat because all the energy in your muscles will have been used up.
- Eat protein (fish, egg or pulses and seeds) within half an hour of exercise to assist with muscle repair and growth.
- Make sure you are properly hydrated. This is essential to weight loss, because fat burning increases levels of toxins in your system which then need to be flushed out by your liver and kidneys. If there isn't adequate water, your body will burn fat less efficiently.

- Make sure you have rest days. If you don't allow your body to recuperate adequately between exercise sessions, you can actually lose muscle tissue. This, in turn, could cause your metabolism to slow down. By letting your body recover properly, you can work to maximum capacity in your next workout and burn yet more fat.

When you start exercising properly, you should quickly start to notice a difference in how you look. Don't forget that muscle weighs more than fat, so even if you don't appear to be losing weight on the scales (see page 87), you will still be making progress. Besides, fluctuations of a few pounds either way are perfectly normal.

Above all, be patient with yourself. If you keep eating healthily, exercising regularly and enjoying your life, your body will eventually settle at a weight that is perfect for you.

CHAPTER 8

YOUR HAIR AND SKIN

My nutritional approach to PCOS will, ultimately, reduce *all* the symptoms of PCOS, including the sometimes very distressing hirsutism and acne. However, improvements can sometimes be rather slow, and it may be up to three months before they become evident.

There are specific skin and hair supplements which can help (see pages 120–22, 124–5), but you may want to discuss other options with your doctor, as some drugs and treatments can make excess hair and acne easier to bear while you are waiting for the effects of the dietary changes to really take effect.

YOUR HAIR

Distressingly, symptoms of PCOS can involve having problems with both excess hair on your face and body and thinning hair on your head at the same time. But don't despair – there are quite a few options for you.

EXCESS HAIR (HIRSUTISM)
PCOS sufferers very commonly experience troublesome excess hair on the chin, upper lip, cheeks, sideburn area, around the nipples, the inside of the thighs and both the upper and lower back.

This hirsutism is driven by the action of male hormones (androgens), so the hair on the arms and legs may become darker and coarser than elsewhere, and may thicken in areas where a man might typically be hairy.

Although this is unlikely to affect physical health in the way that some of the other PCOS symptoms do, it can be extremely distressing, and many patients tell me it affects them psychologically.

Through making the recommended changes to your diet and taking the supplements I suggest, you will be taking huge steps towards controlling your body's production of androgens and this will eventually stem the growth of excess hair. However, it takes about four months for changes in facial hair (which can have the biggest impact on how you feel as a woman) to take effect. So regardless of how much or little excess hair you have, if the problem is affecting your quality of life and relationships, it is important for you to get help while you are waiting for my nutritional solutions to work, which may mean thinking about ways of removing the excess hair.

For direct treatment of hirsutism the choices are:

Bleaching

This does not remove excess hair, but lightens the colour so it appears less obvious. You can buy a home-bleaching kit from a chemist or have your hair bleached at a beauty salon. The effect lasts about four weeks with minimal side effects (although sensitive skin may become temporarily red and irritated).

Shaving/plucking/threading

It is not true that a shaved hair grows back more quickly, but shaving may make the root of the hair thicker, and therefore appear coarser when it does regrow. Shaving is cheap, but will need to be repeated every few days.

Plucking takes the hair out by the root and the effect lasts up to six weeks. It is time consuming and, for some women, may make the hair grow darker and thicker (although some find regrowth is lighter and finer).

Threading originated in the Middle East and is now very popular in the West. Cotton thread is rolled and twisted over the hair to form a series of knots, which pull the hair out by the root. It lasts as long as plucking (two to six weeks), but some believe that over time the technique damages the hair follicle, reducing regrowth. Threading has to be done by a skilled practitioner, but it is relatively inexpensive and now widely available.

Epilators

These can be bought from chemists or electrical stores and are used at home. They are shaped like an electric razor, but have a tweezer head which rotates and pulls the hair out by the root. The effect will last about two to six weeks, much longer than shaving. However, it can be quite painful for those with sensitive skin and the hair has to be quite long (over 0.5cm) before you can epilate.

Waxing

Warm wax is applied to the hair and fabric strips are then put on over the wax and pulled off quickly, taking the hair with them. This can be done at home or in a salon. The effect lasts about two to six weeks. Waxing can cause a rash or redness, but this fades quite quickly. The disadvantages of waxing are that the hair must be relatively long (0.5cm) before it can be re-waxed and the process can sometimes cause discolouration on darker skins.

There is a good organic hair-removal product called MOOM which contains pure essential oils to help feed the skin (see www.natural healthpractice.com under Natural Beauty Products for more information). The chemical-free formula is designed to nourish the skin and the fabric strips can be re-used, making it an environmentally-friendly waxing option.

Topical creams

Depilatory creams are applied to the skin where they dissolve the keratin in the hair. After a few minutes the cream is removed (rinsed or scraped off) along with the hair. These are used at home and the effect can last up to two weeks. The cream does not affect the root, so hair grows back quickly and the creams may irritate sensitive skins.

Another type of cream – Vaniqa (eflornithine hydrochloride) – is available on prescription. It supposedly suppresses hair-follicle activity, but must be used continually and it can take six to eight weeks to see the effects. It may need to be combined with hair-removal techniques, as it does not actually remove the hair. Unfortunately, up to 14 per cent of women who use it experience acne as a consequence – ironic considering it is often prescribed to women with PCOS, most of whom already suffer with acne.

Electrolysis

Even with the advent of lasers, electrolysis is still considered the most permanent way of removing excess hair. The hair is given an 'electric shock' by inserting a fine needle into the hair follicle and applying an electric current. This cuts off the oxygen and blood supply to the hair causing it to die from the root. This is time consuming and can be costly (you may need many sessions over months or years). It can also be quite painful and some redness may occur straight after the treatment, but this fades quite quickly.

Laser

Laser hair removal involves focusing a laser beam on the hair follicles underneath the skin to destroy them and stop the hair from growing.

FINDING A GOOD PRACTITIONER

With electrolysis, laser treatment and IPL you face risks such as burns or changes in the pigmentation of the skin so you should ensure that you find a registered, insured and well-trained practitioner. A helpful website is www.consultingroom.com, which has a list of registered clinics.

It works best on women with dark hair and light skin, as the pigment in the follicle absorbs the laser energy. It is not effective on women with blonde or white facial hair. It's considered an effective way to permanently reduce hair but not to permanently remove it, as many can experience hair regrowth a few years after treatment.

This is not a swift solution – most women need a course of six to eight treatments with four weeks between each one. It is costly and can be painful and there is a possibility of scarring and discolouration of the skin, especially in darker-skinned women.

Intense pulsed light (IPL)

For women with darker skin and fair hair who can't have laser treatment, this may offer a solution. It uses light of various wavelengths to destroy the hair follicle (with the laser only one wavelength is used). It is said to be less painful than laser treatment with reduced risk of scarring. Like the laser treatment, however, it is time consuming and costly. You need six to ten treatments one to three months apart.

HAIR LOSS

Another distressing symptom of PCOS is thinning hair on the scalp. This is called female-pattern hair loss or androgenic alopecia (because it is driven by male hormones). You may experience hair loss if you are more sensitive to the androgens in your system, even if your blood tests show you to have 'normal' androgen levels.

Before you automatically assume PCOS is causing your hair loss you should try to rule out all other possible causes (thyroid problems, iron and other nutrient deficiencies or stress).

By following the dietary recommendations in this book you will reduce your sensitivity to male hormones, but do also ensure you are getting enough protein in your diet. Not only does this contribute to balancing blood-sugar levels (see page 45), but your hair is 80 to 95 per cent protein and a diet low in protein may retard growth or cause hair to thin. Switching your pattern of eating to little and often can also be useful because the energy to form hair cells reduces four hours after eating. By snacking between meals you can help to ensure that the process doesn't stop!

You should be on a programme of supplements for your PCOS (as outlined in Chapter 5), but deficiencies in certain nutrients can make hair loss much worse, so make sure that the supplements you are taking contain good amounts of the following:

Biotin

This nutrient, which is part of the B-vitamin family, helps balance blood sugar (see pages 71–2), but it is also active in reducing hair loss. It is also beneficial for your skin and nails.

Vitamin B12

As well as having a blood test to check your iron stores (see below), I suggest that you are tested for vitamin B12 deficiency as this can cause hair loss (as well as fatigue and mental confusion). Vitamin B12 works alongside iron in the production of red blood cells and the trans-portation of oxygen in the bloodstream. Testing for vitamin B12 is particularly important if you have been taking metformin as it can cause vitamin B12 deficiency.[1]

Omega 3 fish oils

Fish oils can prevent your hair from drying out and breaking, so make sure you take an Omega 3 fish-oil supplement with at least 770mg EPA and 510mg DHA. If you are vegetarian you can use flaxseed oil (1,000mg).

Horsetail (Equisetum arvense)

Horsetail is a herb which has a high silica content. Silica forms part of all connective tissue which includes not only your hair, but also your nails and skin. It can help to strengthen hair and promote its growth, as well as improving its quality. Take 300mg two to three times daily.

Iron

If you are experiencing hair loss or thinning, ask your doctor to check your ferritin levels. When you are tested for anaemia, the lab measures the level of iron available in your red blood cells (haemoglobin). However, iron is also stored as ferritin in other parts of the body, such

PRACTICAL TIPS FOR PREVENTING HAIR LOSS

- Don't brush too vigorously as this causes your hair to break.
- Use a wide-toothed comb, especially after washing, so you don't have to pull at your hair to untangle it.
- Avoid tight ponytails or braiding which can put strain on your hair and make it break more easily.
- Enrich your hair by rubbing in oil, so it is completely soaked (olive oil or coconut oil work particularly well). Cover with a shower cap and either leave on for the evening or overnight. To remove the oil, put shampoo directly on to your hair and rub in before wetting.

as the spleen and liver. Your ferritin level should be over 70ng/ml. If it is lower than this, you should take an iron supplement. You need adequate levels of vitamin C for your body to effectively absorb iron, so for maximum absorption take 500mg of vitamin C with your iron supplement on an empty stomach. Avoid taking iron at the same time of day as other supplements as it can block the uptake of other minerals such as zinc.

Avoid taking iron in the form of ferrous sulphate (also called iron sulphate), which is less easily absorbed by the body. Only 2–10 per cent of the iron from this type of iron supplement is actually absorbed by your body, and even then, half is eliminated, causing blackening of your stools and constipation. Ferrous sulphate is classed as an inorganic iron. Organic irons are much more easily absorbed and do not affect the bowels in same way. Look for iron in the form of ascorbates or citrates (see iron supplements on www.naturalhealthpractice.com or see Useful Resources, page 217).

Try to avoid drinking regular black tea with your meals as this can block the uptake of iron from your food. Similarly, the phosphates found in fizzy soft drinks can prevent iron from being absorbed by the body. Herbal teas and diluted fruit juices are fine.

Lysine

The amino acid lysine is particularly helpful for reducing hair loss as it plays a part in the absorption of iron. This amino acid is even more important if you have low iron (ferritin) stores (see above) as it is thought that for some women ferritin levels do not improve even with iron supplementation unless they have adequate supplies of lysine.[2] Take 500–1,000mg daily.

Drug treatment

Your doctor may offer you minoxidil (also known as Regaine) to apply to your hair. This acts as a vasodilator, widening blood vessels so that more blood can carry nutrients and oxygen to the hair follicles. Side effects can include burning or irritation of the eyes and itching and redness of the scalp. One unfortunate side effect for women with PCOS is that it can cause unwanted hair growth elsewhere on the body. Also, be warned that in some cases, minoxidil can actually trigger more hair loss without regrowth.

YOUR SKIN

PCOS can trigger acne, skin tags (known as acrochordons) and skin discolouration (acanthosis nigricans) in some women. My dietary recommendations and supplement programme will certainly help to control the excess production of male hormones which may well be affecting your skin. But while these lifestyle changes improve your underlying physiology, there are other treatments you can try in the interim.

ACNE
Acne is thought to be a combination of four factors:

- Increased sebum (oil) production
- Obstructed hair follicles
- Colonization of bacteria
- Inflammation

Increased sebum (oil) production: Sebum is produced by the sebaceous glands in the skin. These are attached to the hair follicles and lubricate your skin and hair. Male hormones appear to trigger an increase in sebum production, but you don't necessarily have to have high levels of male hormones to be affected. In some women, the sebaceous glands in the skin seem to be more sensitive to androgens.

Obstructed hair follicles: Excess sebum mixes with dead skin cells (keratin) and ends up trapped in the pores. Normally skin cells grow, die and are shed, but when you have acne the cells become sticky and plug up the hair follicles, causing blackheads and whiteheads.

Colonization of bacteria: We all have bacteria on the skin, known as Propionibacteria acnes, but if you have acne you probably have more of these bacteria, and your immune system will set up an inflammatory reaction to deal with the invaders.

Inflammation: The response of the immune system is to cause redness, tenderness and irritation, resulting in red bumps and pustules.

Natural treatments

Before talking to your doctor, ensure your programme of supplements contains adequate quantities of the following:

- **Zinc:** This is an important mineral for your skin and it is also crucial for PCOS in general. If you are suffering with acne, I suggest you take an extra zinc supplement (15mg) in addition to the zinc in your multivitamin and mineral capsule. Take it last thing at night on an empty stomach. Normally, it is best to take supplements with food because they are 'supplementary' to what you are eating, but with skin problems the extra zinc works best when taken just before bed.

- **Tea tree oil:** This essential oil has both anti-bacterial and anti-fungal properties, so can be very helpful for acne. Use it on the skin in a diluted form: a 5 per cent solution of tea tree oil has been shown to be as effective as a 5 per cent solution of one of the most common over-the-counter remedies for acne, benzoyl peroxide. It does, however, take longer to work.[3]

- **Aloe vera:** Aloe vera can be used on your skin for acne. Try to get a gel that contains few preservatives and has a high aloe vera content. It can be effective in lessening redness, swelling and inflammation and can heal damaged skin and old acne scar tissue. Aloe vera also has anti-bacterial benefits and acts as an astringent. Apply it to affected areas.

- **Agnus castus:** This balancing herb can also be helpful, especially if your acne gets worse with your menstrual cycle (even if your cycle is erratic). See page 81 for more on agnus castus and dosage.
- **Echinacea:** This immune-strengthening herb can be useful for treating acne as it will help your body control any bacterial overgrowth. Take one teaspoon of tincture in a little water, two or three times daily, or take 300–400mg in capsule form, twice daily.
- **Omega 3 oils:** It might sound strange to use more oils for a problem that is caused by too much oil (sebum), but the Omega 3s have such great anti-inflammatory properties they can only do good. If you are already following the dietary advice and supplements programme, this will be included in your diet already. See page 75 for dosage.
- **Probiotics:** Make sure you are taking a good probiotic as 70 per cent of your immune function is in your gut. This means that these beneficial bacteria in your digestive system can help to control not only inflammation, but also negative bacteria and yeasts. Again, if you are following my supplements programme, you will already have a probiotic in your diet.

Medical treatments

If your skin is very bad, your GP may suggest you try the Pill (particularly one brand called Dianette), which has an effect on male hormones. You may, alternatively, be offered a number of different creams and drugs.

I recommend trying the nutritional advice in this book first, together with natural remedies like aloe vera, to address your skin problems, and use a good mineral make-up or concealer to cover your skin while you wait for your hormones to correct. If, after this, you still find your acne is affecting your emotional wellbeing, there is nothing wrong with exploring the medical options. Start with benzoyl peroxide, though, which is a milder treatment, and only move up the list of stronger treatments if you need to.

- **Benzoyl peroxide:** This is a frequently used medical treatment for acne. It is available from chemists in varying strengths or from your GP. It works by introducing oxygen into the pores which stops the Propionibacteria from surviving (the bacteria are anaerobic and die in the presence of oxygen). It also helps to clear the follicle of dead skin cells, so preventing the pores from becoming blocked. Side effects can include dry and flaking skin, redness and burning.
- **Antibiotics:** Your doctor can prescribe topical antibiotics, but it seems that women with PCOS do not have much success with these.[4] Oral antibiotics such as tetracyclines work by managing the overgrowth of bacteria which, in turn, controls the inflammation in the skin.

  Tetracycline is the most prescribed antibiotic for acne, but should not be used if you are pregnant (do tell your doctor if you are trying to conceive). Erythromycin is another antibiotic used for acne. The drug information suggests it can be used in pregnancy.

  Unfortunately, all antibiotics carry possible side effects such as stomach upset and nausea. Oral antibiotics also do not discriminate between 'good' and 'bad' bacteria and will inevitably wipe out the beneficial bacteria in your gut as well as the bad. This can cause a vaginal yeast (candida) infection.

If you do take an antibiotic, make sure you are also taking a good probiotic supplement (not a probiotic drink) at a different time of day.

- **Topical retinoids:** These are derivatives of vitamin A applied in the form of a cream. They work by preventing skin cells from clogging up the hair follicles.

- **Oral isotretinoin (also called Roaccutane):** This is also a derivative of vitamin A and is very effective at decreasing the production of sebum. But it carries a number of possible side effects such as dry skin, joint pains, stomach and bowel discomfort, nausea, fatigue and thinning hair. It can also cause changes in behaviour, depressed mood, hallucinations and sleep problems.

It is very important not to become pregnant while taking this drug as it carries a very high risk of severe birth defects, even if the woman has only been taking the drug for a short period of time.

SKIN TAGS (ACROCHORDONS)

These are floppy pieces of skin which can often be found around the neck, armpits, eyelids, chest and groin. They are usually benign and are linked to insulin resistance. Skin tags can be removed by surgery or they can be frozen or lasered off, but they may grow back if the underlying cause – insulin resistance – is not addressed.

I recommend that you stick to my PCOS dietary plan (see Chapter 4) for three months before talking to anyone about having your skin tags removed. That way your insulin resistance should be in check, and so there will be less chance of the tags growing back.

SKIN DISCOLOURATION (ACANTHOSIS NIGRICANS)

This is also often caused by insulin resistance. There is nothing you can do to treat the discolouration directly, but if you follow my dietary recommendations (see Chapter 4), you should see any dark areas on your skin start to lighten. In the meantime, use good make-up or concealer to boost your confidence – try to choose the most natural product available to prevent your body from dealing with too many chemicals (see pages 150–51).

SPIRONOLACTONE

This drug is often prescribed to women with PCOS who have problems with their skin and hair. It is an 'anti-androgen', and although it has been prescribed for reducing hair growth, improving hair loss and also acne for over twenty years, it is not actually licensed for that use. (It is a diuretic used for treating fluid retention.)

Side effects of spironolactone can include fatigue, nausea, breast tenderness and dizziness and menstrual irregularity – which means it's not a great treatment for PCOS – and research using it on hair loss has shown that it is not spectacularly successful.[5] Think carefully before you choose to try it.

CHAPTER 9

STRESS AND PCOS

In this chapter I will analyse the impact of stress on your PCOS symptoms and give practical advice about managing – and hopefully reducing – the stress in your life.

For many women, the PCOS symptoms of weight gain, acne and excess hair leave them feeling depressed and anxious. But physical wellness often goes hand in hand with emotional wellness, so by lessening stress and addressing psychological issues, you can then concentrate more on your diet and lifestyle changes and getting the better of those erratic hormones.

STRESS MAKES PCOS WORSE

Even if you're the most relaxed woman in the world, the stress hormones (adrenaline and cortisol) in your system will be contributing to your PCOS symptoms. These two hormones rise and fall depending on what and how you eat and according to the dips and troughs of your blood-sugar rollercoaster. On a poor diet, your blood sugar is likely to undulate throughout the day, causing the body to release cortisol, which triggers the release of more insulin, which then targets your ovaries, stimulating them to produce more testosterone (which makes the PCOS symptoms so much worse).

By simply switching to a healthy diet (see Chapter 4) you will be helping to control the release of these stress hormones and diminishing the intensity of your PCOS symptoms.

However, this is only part of the stress picture. Most of us have much less control over outside stresses – deadlines, rude people, debt, not enough sleep. There are so many things that can stress you and trigger the release of stress hormones – so antagonizing your PCOS.

Our reaction to stress is very individual because it is the perception of stress rather than the stress itself that has the biggest impact on mental and physical health. Dr Selye, known as 'the grandfather of stress' and author of *The Stress of Life*[1] said:

> No one can live without experiencing some degree of stress all the time. You may think that only serious disease or intensive physical or mental injury can cause stress. This is false. Crossing a busy intersection, exposure to a draught, or even sheer joy are enough to activate the body's stress mechanisms to some extent. Stress is not even necessarily bad for you; it is also the spice of life, for any emotion, any activity causes stress. But, of course, your system must be prepared to take it. The same stress which makes one person sick can be an invigorating experience for another.

If you have PCOS, your body will most likely find it hard to deal with stress and will be more sensitive to it than most women's,[2] and you could end up producing more cortisol, which can increase the levels of male hormones.[3]

Adrenaline and cortisol are called your 'fight-or-flight' hormones – they are normally released when your life is in danger. Adrenaline gets you focused and alert and cortisol increases levels of sugar and fat in your bloodstream, so you can run or fight for your life. If you live under chronic stress – as so many of us do these days – these hormones will be active and doing their best to prepare you for an almost constant fight-or-flight situation. This is unhealthy for anyone, but for women with PCOS, it causes a catalogue of problems when they then have to also factor in the emotional stresses of dealing with PCOS on a daily basis. And layer upon layer of stress definitely makes PCOS worse.

If you carry more weight around the middle of your body (as many PCOS sufferers do), studies show you are very likely to produce more cortisol when stressed.[4] The problem is that stress can make you eat more: after it pumps out all those hormones to help you deal with what it thinks is going to be 'fight or flight', your body sends out instructions for you to 'refuel', so you can stock up reserves ready for some future attack. You'll feel this as an increase in appetite and strong cravings for foods containing carbohydrates and fat (such as chocolate and cakes for instance). This can lead to comfort eating and even bingeing.[5]

Unless you have actually been running or fighting for your life, any extra food you eat now will not be used up, but will be deposited, stubbornly, as fat – very often around your middle.

Another way that stress makes PCOS worse is through its effect on the adrenal glands. Normally, the adrenal glands pump out an andro-gen (a male hormone) called androstenedione which a healthy body converts to oestrogen. But when you are under stress androstenedione is converted instead to testosterone.

We know that stress can affect fertility. Some women notice their periods stop if they are going through a traumatic time, so there is no doubt that stress plays a destructive role on the delicate PCOS hormonal balance. Stress alone can also cause hair loss and thinning and increase the possibility of flare-ups with acne, making your strug-gle with PCOS tougher to control.

BREAK THE STRESS EFFECT

If you want to stop stress from making your PCOS worse, my strongest recommendation is that you balance your blood-sugar levels, and consider taking a combination of herbs and supplements known to ease the effects of stress.

BALANCING BLOOD SUGAR

It has never been more important to follow my dietary recommendations in Chapter 4. In particular, making the switch to unrefined carbohydrates and eating every three hours are vital measures because they will stop stress hormones being released as a result of blood-sugar swings. Many of my patients say this really helps them cope, even if there's nothing they can do to control the stresses outside their lives.

Just sorting out your blood sugar allows you to take a step back and look at your problems in a more detached way, rather than feeling permanently overwhelmed.

As an added bonus, controlling your blood-sugar swings could also mean that you are able to prevent the following potentially stressful emotional consequences:

- Irritability
- Fatigue
- Aggressive outbursts
- Depression
- Palpitations
- Mood swings
- Forgetfulness
- Anxiety
- Confusion
- Inability to concentrate

- Panic attacks
- Crying spells
- Headaches/migraines
- Food cravings
- Digestive problems like bloating, flatulence
- Lack of sex drive

STRESS-BUSTING SUPPLEMENTS

Ensure that you are taking the supplements and herbs you need (see Chapter 5). Chromium and the B vitamins are particularly useful in smoothing out the body's stress response, and Siberian ginseng and magnesium are worth taking. (In my clinics, I use a supplement called Tranquil Woman which may be useful. It is available from health food stores or www.naturalhealthpractice.com.)

PRACTICAL WAYS TO REDUCE STRESS

So many women say they no longer have any time for themselves as they are always trying to fit so much in to their lives.

We have machines to do our washing and dishwashing, food and clothes can be delivered to our door, yet we seem to have less time than we did a generation ago. Technology often makes things worse because mobile phones, texts and email mean we are always reachable and can never seem to escape. The social network sites add to the problem if you become addicted to the minutiae of everyday life and feel stressed if you don't 'check in' regularly.

With this information overload and the constant demands on your time, it's really vital – particularly if you have PCOS – to carve out some space for yourself to relax and unwind. Here are some tips to help you do just that.

TAKE WARM BATHS

Set aside time at the end of the day for a warm, relaxing bath. It is all too easy to try to fit in a couple of emails just before going to bed and, before you know it, you're sucked in to spending an hour on the computer. Be strict with yourself and have a definite cut-off when you go for a bath. Turn down the lighting, play some relaxing music, put one to two drops of aromatherapy oils in the water (lavender or ylang-ylang) and soak for about twenty minutes.

A massage with aromatherapy oils is also a good way to relax, and always carry a tissue with two drops of lavender or lemon essential oil on it to inhale as and when you need it.

GIVE YOUR MIND A BREAK

Set aside ten to fifteen minutes every day to stop thinking. Call it meditation if you like, but just use it as a daily opportunity to stop the thoughts and internal dialogue from going round and round in your head. Find the time of day that works best for you – often it can be early in the morning or just before bed.

Find a comfortable place to sit (a chair is fine). Then close your eyes and just let your body relax. The easiest way to start is to focus on your breathing: take a few deep breaths, releasing any tension, and think about breathing in and out. Try playing some soothing music or imagining yourself in a beautiful garden.

If your thoughts start to take over, bring your mind back to your breathing. Or try muscle relaxation to focus your mind on something and stop it thinking: the aim is to tense each part of your body in turn as you breathe in, hold the breath for five seconds and then relax the muscles and breathe out for ten seconds. You can either start at your head, screwing up your eyes and forehead first and then working down your body or start at your toes and work up. Either way is good. You may find it hard to sit still at first and only manage five minutes, but that is fine. Quite soon you'll be able to sit for up to ten minutes.

Relaxation will also help you to lose weight (see page 106). Research shows that women who use relaxation techniques like meditation, positive visualization and yoga have sustained weight loss compared to women who follow calorie restriction alone. The reduction in stress levels resulted in women who felt happier and healthier and no longer craved sweet or fatty foods.[6]

One particular meditation technique is called mindfulness-based cognitive therapy and is endorsed by NICE and the National Institutes for Health in the US. It has been shown to help improve wellbeing and levels of happiness and to be as effective as drugs for treating depression.[7]

TAKE TIME TO SLEEP

You must ensure that you are sleeping well, not just for your general health and weight (see page 99), but because sleep is crucial in reducing stress levels. Your body registers lack of sleep as a stress in itself, so you will feel worse still if you are not getting enough sleep.

Lack of sleep will increase your levels of cortisol, exacerbating PCOS symptoms and increasing insulin resistance.[8] Cortisol follows a diurnal (daily) rhythm: it should be high in the morning when you wake ready to start the day and it reduces as the day goes on, reaching a low point as you go to sleep. But if you are sleep deprived, you can end up with raised cortisol levels in the afternoon and evening and impaired glucose tolerance which increases insulin resistance.

Don't ever fall into the trap of cutting short your sleep time to fit more into your life. You will get more done – and more efficiently – if you are well rested.

Follow the tips for a good night's sleep on pages 99–101.

EXERCISE

Exercise is crucial for your general health and also in the battle to control PCOS (see Chapter 7), but it is also vital for stress reduction. Stress hormones are designed to be released in tandem with some sort of physical action (you are supposed to be running or fighting for your life), but most modern stress is highly inactive.

By exercising regularly (thirty minutes a day), you will be allowing your body to release those stress hormones before they have a chance to exert a negative effect on your health. Exercise also encourages the release of endorphins which make you feel happier, and it helps reduce anxiety and lifts your self-esteem.

ENJOY YOURSELF

Laughter is supposed to be the best medicine, so make sure you give yourself time to do the things you enjoy. Have fun! This will work towards reducing your stress hormones.

BREATHE PROPERLY

Many people breathe from the top of their chest (shallow breathing). It is a very common consequence of hours spent hunched over a computer or desk and is the same kind of breathing you do when stressed, so doing it without thinking will increase that effect. Try to breathe from lower down – from your diaphragm (belly breathing). This has a relaxing effect on the body. Research by Harvard University has found that breathing slowly and deeply from the stomach significantly reduces stress and anxiety.[9]

Try the following:

- Place your hands over your belly.
- As you breathe in, push your belly out – you should be able to feel your hands being pushed out.
- Pause for a moment.
- Breathe out slowly through your nose.
- As you breathe out, imagine all the tension and stress leaving your body, just like a soft, flowing stream.
- Repeat this ten times and try to do it every day, if possible.

HAVE A HUG

Cuddling can help you feel more relaxed because it reduces the stress hormones and also releases oxytocin.[10] Oxytocin is the hormone released by the pituitary gland during hugging, orgasm and also during labour and breastfeeding. It is also thought to be the hormone released when people are in love; it increases trust and reduces fear.

SORT OUT YOUR PRIORITIES

If you want to beat your PCOS, you *must* make your health your number-one priority and do whatever you can to get a sense of control over your life.

This is likely to mean you'll need to say 'no' a bit more often. You may even need to reassess your job if it is too stressful and requires you to work long hours with little time to eat properly or take any exercise.

If you are the sort who puts yourself under pressure to get 'everything right', now might be a good time to look at your attitude to life in general and perhaps to stop being quite so hard on yourself.

You need to try to take control of your time. What about planning the weekly meals upfront, so you do not have to think about what you are having for dinner each night?

Set up a 'to-do' list and put everything in priority order – this is particularly useful if you tend to sit awake at night going over everything you have to do in your mind. If you've written a list, it's all catalogued, and you can simply remind yourself that there's no need to worry.

ENJOY YOUR FOOD

When you eat, take time to sit down and eat calmly. Many of my patients tell me they eat standing up (particularly breakfast), grabbing mouthfuls of something, while trying to get ready. Instead, try to practise 'mindful eating', so that you are aware of your food, the texture and flavour, for example, rather than eating mindlessly. Put your cutlery down between mouthfuls and enjoy every bite. Eat in a relaxed way, chew your food well and think of your food as the nourishment and fuel that is going to get you through the day.

EMOTIONAL ISSUES

Having PCOS is very likely to throw up for you a number of emotional issues that other women will not experience. Being unhappy with your body image (weight, excess hair and acne) can knock your self-esteem and confidence, and this can affect your relationships with friends, family and partners.

Rest assured, it's not just you. It is now widely acknowledged that PCOS affects you both physically and mentally. Research shows it is common to feel depressed and anxious.[11] You just need to learn how to deal with those feelings and turn the negatives into positives.

It is hardly surprising that you feel bad when what is happening to your body seems to be out of your control, but reading this book, and understanding just what is going on – and all the steps you can take to change it – can make a big difference to how you feel mentally.

As you follow the natural solutions in this book you will notice psychological as well as physical improvements. Your mind and body are so closely interconnected that as you get positive changes in one area you will start to see progress in others and this will put you into a wonderfully positive upward spiral.

Here are some tips and techniques to help put you in a more positive mindset.

CHANGE YOUR INNER DIALOGUE

It is very important to think about how you talk to yourself. Are all your thoughts about yourself negative? Do you tend to think, 'Why I am so fat?' and 'Why am I no good at my job?'

If you ask these sorts of questions, your mind will try and find answers. And if the questions are worded negatively, the answers will inevitably be negative too: 'Because you are lazy and eat too much' or 'Because you are useless'. This then reinforces the negative perception you have of yourself and so the vicious cycle continues.

Try turning this on its head and ask different questions: 'How can I lose weight?' and, 'How can I do this job better?' Your mind will do its best to come up with answers, but this time they are much more likely to be positive: 'You can eat more healthily and start exercising' and 'You could ask if you can go on a training course to get more knowledge to assist you in your job'.

Always give yourself the benefit of the doubt. This is so important if you are going to battle effectively the psychological demons of PCOS. You would always try to forgive a friend if they made a mistake, so do the same with yourself rather than beating yourself up.

Your mind is very powerful – it's up to you to decide whether you want it to help or hinder you.

ACCEPT WHO YOU ARE

We are all unique. There is no one else like you on this planet. So celebrate those differences and accept who you are. It doesn't mean you should stop striving to improve your wellbeing (physically and emotionally), but it does mean accepting that some things you just can't change. In the words of the famous theologian Reinhold Niebuhr: 'Grant me the serenity to accept the things I cannot change, the courage to change the things I can and the wisdom to know the difference.'

LOVE YOURSELF

You need to love and like yourself so that others find you warm, approachable and attractive. What you radiate out is what you get back.

PCOS can really knock you down, so if you're not careful, you can end up believing that you are not good enough, or don't deserve happiness or a successful relationship.

Choose your friends wisely because some may not have your best interests at heart and some may, even unconsciously, try to boost their own confidence by belittling you.

Make a point of surrounding yourself with people who have your best interests at heart, make the changes to your life I recommend in this book and start to believe in yourself.

BE PATIENT WITH YOURSELF

We all want a quick fix, but health, and particularly weight loss, do not work like that. Be patient. My natural solutions are not instant wonders, and if your body takes a while to respond, then that is simply the natural time it needs to heal itself.

Do not be hard on yourself if you don't always follow my recommendations to the letter – look upon them as forever lifestyle changes that you incorporate 80 per cent of the time, and the more gradually the changes take place, the more likely they are to be permanent.

SET SMALL GOALS

Make a list of small goals to keep you motivated. It is far better to have more modest objectives that you can achieve than to promise yourself the impossible. For example, set yourself a target to exercise for thirty minutes a day. That could mean going to the gym, but it could also be a walk at lunchtime. It all counts! Or if you find cutting out alcohol too tough, try saving it just for the weekends. Say no to chocolate, but keep a small bag of fruit or nuts/seeds with you at all times so you won't be tempted to go crazy and make a bad food choice if your blood sugar dips.

REALIZE THAT YOU ARE NOT ALONE

There are many women who feel insecure because of their symptoms, particularly the outwardly visible ones. This is made more difficult by the media bombarding us with images of perfect-looking celebrities (many of whom have spent hours in make-up or have been airbrushed to oblivion). Feeling paranoid about how you look can cause you to put up an invisible barrier without you even realizing it, preventing friends and family from supporting you and making you feel isolated. Share your feelings with other people and let them help you.

EMOTIONAL EATING

So often we eat not because we're hungry but because we're bored, stressed, lonely, depressed or tired, which leads not only to eating the wrong foods, but also to overeating, because whatever we put in our mouths simply doesn't satisfy. This can commonly contribute to the characteristic weight gain of PCOS.

Here are a few tips and techniques for avoiding the pitfalls of emotional eating:

- Hypnotherapy (see page 143) can be helpful, so if emotional eating is something you struggle with, do consider seeing a professional for this.
- Be aware of your eating triggers as this is the best way to break bad habits.
- After a binge, ask yourself: 'Was it worth it?' How did the guilt affect you? And just before the next stress-induced binge ask yourself: 'Is this going to help me? Do I really need to eat this?' Pause for a few seconds as you open the fridge or cupboard. Turn mindless eating into mindful eating.
- If you do have a tendency to binge eat, try to become aware of what you are eating – the smell, texture, taste – and you will find that you will eat less and retrain your body and mind to think differently about not only how much, but also what you eat.

- Cravings typically last for ten minutes, so recognize this and try to divert your mind and ride them out. Distract yourself by phoning a friend, reading a book or going for a walk. But if distraction doesn't work, don't deny a craving – it is better to have one piece of organic dark chocolate now than to end up with an urge so strong that you eat the whole bar.

- The best snack to beat a craving is a handful of nuts (six walnuts, twelve almonds or twenty peanuts) with two glasses of water. But never eat out of a bag or container. Always put food on a plate or in a bowl, so you can see exactly how much you're eating. Divide a 282g (10oz) packet of nuts into ten small plastic bags. Make sure you eat only one bag at a sitting and put the rest away where you can't see them.

- Don't shop on an empty stomach. Shopping when you are hungry makes you far more likely to crave calorie-rich, sugary, fatty foods.

- Make a list of exactly what you need when shopping and stick to it.

- Try changing your routine. Habit can affect a craving, so shake up what you do, even if it's just slightly. Move your desk, sit differently, get up every so often and stretch or drink water. Walk a different route to work so that you avoid passing that bakery or sweet shop.

- Drinking a glass of water before you eat can curb a food craving by making you feel slightly full. Water can also have a direct impact on energy – you may be reaching for a sugar fix when what you really need is rehydration.

- Stock your kitchen with healthy snacks. This will reduce the temptation to go for unhealthy foods – after all, you are less likely to put your coat on at 9pm to go out and buy something.

- If you enjoy the ritual of sitting down and having something to eat, spread a piece of wholemeal toast with organic peanut butter and pure fruit jam. You may be surprised at what will satisfy the craving and it is a far healthier option than sitting down with a packet of white-flour-and-sugar biscuits.

- Keep a food diary. It definitely works. Much of your eating is done unconsciously, and writing it down can make you more aware of your food choices. This, in itself, can prompt you to make healthier decisions.

GETTING PROFESSIONAL HELP
If you've been living with PCOS for many years, some of your patterns of thinking may have become ingrained, particularly when it comes to food, and you may need professional help to change them.

Cognitive behavioural therapy (CBT)
CBT can be a very effective way of changing the way you think and altering your behaviour. It works with the conscious mind to teach you to recognize the negative thinking patterns that are making you depressed and anxious. If you can change your thoughts, very often your feelings and behaviour will change too. CBT can also help you to see the triggers of comfort eating and provide you with tools to stop these negative thoughts and habits.

CBT has been used with women with PCOS, not only for depression, but also (combined with nutrition and diet) for support with weight loss.[12]

Hypnotherapy
This is very useful for boosting self-esteem and confidence. Hypnotherapy works on the premise that there are two states of consciousness – the conscious and the subconscious – which may be at odds with each other. For example, a woman may say that she wants a baby, but her subconscious fears may be stopping her from getting pregnant.

Hypnotherapy enables communication with the subconscious where habits tend to be stored. It can also change the sort of habitual negative thinking that can trigger depression, low self-esteem and lack of willpower and it can give you the necessary motivation to begin to love your own body and take care of it – which is particularly important if you have PCOS.

So if you find yourself eating when you are not hungry, but using food to fill a void, hypnotherapy could be useful. It can give you the willpower to eat healthily and exercise and to turn away foods high in sugar, saturated fat and refined carbohydrates. It can help you to feel fuller quicker, eat more slowly and eat less than ever before.

Hypnotherapy isn't for everyone, but it can work for some people, especially those who have for years been reaching for food when they know they aren't hungry. It aims to give you control back over your thoughts and behaviours.

If you can find a practitioner who combines hypnotherapy with NLP (neurolinguistic programming) this can be even more powerful. NLP uses the power of the mind and language to change the way you think and to break old habits which may be holding you back.

Counselling

Some of your patterns and attitudes around food may be rooted in your childhood. Perhaps you were brought up to finish everything on your plate and now find it difficult to leave anything because it seems wasteful. You might have been given sweets as a treat or for being good and now see food as a reward. Counselling can show you that you are not controlled by your past and you can learn to let it go and form a new set of healthy attitudes and patterns.

Counselling or any 'talking therapy' can make you aware of conditioned patterns. Counsellors do not give advice, but are often able to see things more clearly and from a different perspective. Because they are not friends or family members it means that you can tell them anything without being judged and in complete confidence. This gives you the opportunity to discuss emotions that you may have bottled up, such as anxiety, anger at having PCOS ('Why me?'), problems with relationships, feelings of worthlessness, maybe grief because you have not conceived. Exploring these issues safely and securely with a trained counsellor can provide a huge relief, ease stress and, ultimately, help you to control your PCOS symptoms.

Support groups

There is a wonderful PCOS charity in the UK called Verity (www.verity-pcos.org.uk) that organizes talks, so you can meet up with like-minded women. There are also brilliant discussion groups on their website. It is much easier to stay on track and keep motivated when you know that you are not alone and that other women are thinking the same thoughts and going through the same experiences as you.

CHAPTER 10

ENVIRONMENTAL HORMONE DISRUPTORS

When you have PCOS, your body has to try to cope with unfamiliar balances of hormones produced as a consequence of your insulin resistance and misaligned monthly cycle. This can make you hypersensitive to the slightest chemical changes both internally (from the food you eat) and externally (on the skin and in the air you breathe).

Studies show that outside chemicals really can affect the delicate balance of your hormones, and PCOS sufferers are particularly sensitive to this.

I recommend my patients do whatever they can to reduce the toxic load on their system while they are working to take control of their PCOS. This means trying to avoid – as much as possible – the toxins so commonly used in household products like cleaning fluids and toiletries and the plastic in bottles and containers.

In previous chapters we looked at how your diet, exercise and stress levels and emotions can affect PCOS symptoms. But you should also be aware that things like washing-up liquid or your body lotion could also be making your symptoms worse.

Commonly used chemicals can disrupt your hormones by interfering with their production or utilization or by mimicking their action.

When it comes to PCOS, they can make things worse by making one particular hormone (perhaps oestrogen) more dominant or sometimes, by stopping your body from using your hormones effectively (exacerbating insulin resistance).

These chemicals are defined as substances that can 'interfere with the synthesis, secretion, transport, binding, action, or elimination of natural hormones in the body that are responsible for development, behaviour, fertility, and maintenance of homeostasis (normal cell metabolism)'.[1] Experts know them by a number of different names, including:

- environmental hormone disruptors
- endocrine disruptor chemicals (EDCs)
- xenoestrogens (meaning 'foreign' oestrogens)
- hormone mimics or blockers.

The problem is that these chemicals are everywhere. They are found in plastics, pesticides, hormone medications like the Pill and HRT (residues end up in your water supply), dental fillings, till and credit card receipts, the resins coating the inside of food and drink cans, toiletries, cosmetics, lipsticks, perfumes, hairspray, nail polish, toothpaste, spermicides, deodorants and body washes.

The Government would probably like us to believe that these chemicals are perfectly safe, but there is a growing body of evidence to suggest that they are not. DEFRA (the Government's Department for Environment, Food and Rural Affairs) has even pointed out that one third of the male fish in the UK's rivers are becoming feminized by chemical residues in their water.

But although we are clearly seeing the impact of these chemicals on wildlife, it is not always easy to link them to humans and to be specific about their effects on our general and reproductive health.

The Endocrine Society in America (which deals with issues concerning hormones) released a scientific statement in 2009 saying these chemicals *do* have effects on male and female reproduction, various cancers, thyroid function, metabolism and obesity and heart health.[2]

Chemicals can influence every system in our bodies. They can affect ovulation and increase our risk of hormonally driven problems (which is why they should be avoided, if possible, if you have PCOS), but they also cause infertility by reducing quality and quantity of sperm in men, pushing young girls through puberty earlier and creating malformations in male babies such as hypospadias (where the opening of the urethra is down the shaft of the penis instead of at the top) and undescended testes.

There is certainly enough evidence to suggest that these chemicals have widespread effects on our health, regardless of age or gender – but if you have PCOS you are likely to be particularly vulnerable.

One chemical, bisphenol A (BPA), which is used in the manufacture of plastic, has been linked to an increased risk of PCOS[3] and of miscarriage.[4] The blood levels of BPA in women with PCOS is significantly higher than in those without the condition and also is associated with higher levels of testosterone and insulin resistance.[5] Other research has found that exposing rats to BPA early in life gives them PCOS in adulthood.[6]

We know that these chemicals can damage the follicles in the ovaries,[7] stop them from functioning normally and also stop the maturation of eggs in the follicles.[8] There is also research suggesting the chemicals could increase the risk of Type 2 diabetes.[9]

Other research has shown that low-dose exposure to the chemicals can increase the chances of being overweight and insulin resistance in non-diabetics.[10]

Even low doses of chemicals like these can affect us because they can still interact with hormone receptors and stop hormones working properly. Because, very often, they act like hormones themselves they can easily throw our delicately balanced hormone systems out of kilter.

More worrying is the fact that some chemicals are fat loving (lipophilic), which means they stay in our fat stores and cause problems long after we have been around them.

REDUCING YOUR EXPOSURE

In the modern world, we are typically exposed to many different kinds of chemicals every single day. No one knows what the combined effect of this cocktail is on our health, but it is clear that it is particularly important for you to avoid them as far as possible, if you are trying to manage a condition like PCOS.

You won't be able to escape contact with these chemicals completely, but there are certain choices you can make that will limit your exposure:

YOUR SKIN

Your skin is extremely porous, and chemicals can be very easily absorbed through it – up to 60 per cent of what you put on your skin, in fact. (This is why nicotine and HRT patches work so well.) It is estimated that over the course of a day you could be exposing yourself to around 500 different synthetic chemicals through your skin alone – and women can ingest more than 4lb (2kg) of lipstick in a lifetime, both swallowed and absorbed through the lining of the mouth. (Long-lasting lipsticks are worse because they contain plastics and nylon which glues the colour to the lips.)

It is a good idea to try to avoid toiletries, cosmetics, shampoos, moisturizers which list any of the words below in their ingredients:

- Parabens (e.g. methylparabens)
- Phthalates
- Talc
- Triclosan

- Surfactants
- Synthetic fragrances (parfum)
- Formaldehyde
- BHT
- DEA, MEA, TEA
- Polyethylene glycol
- Propylene glycol
- Sodium lauryl (laureth) sulphate
- Colourants
- Petrochemicals
- Urea
- Butylphenyl, Methylpropional

This may look daunting, but I believe you shouldn't put anything on your skin that you would not be prepared to eat.

Also, there are many products that claim they are 'natural' and are not. If you are confused, go to www.naturalhealthpractice.com and look under 'Natural Beauty Products' as I have checked the labels of many different products to show you which ones are safe to use. Health shops are a good place to source natural products; and they are increasingly appearing in mainstream chemists and supermarkets too, but always check the labels carefully.

To anyone with PCOS, I'd recommend using natural soaps on their body, oils and balms for their skin and to add aromatherapy oils like lavender, ylang-ylang and rose to the bath instead of chemically laden products. (Remember, in a bath you are soaking in those chemicals for some time and they will seep through your skin fairly easily.)

YOUR FOOD

You can significantly reduce your exposure to pesticides, insecticides and fungicides by buying organic food where possible. It's estimated that around 3,900 different brands of pesticides are used on food or in homes. Some fruit and vegetables can be sprayed ten times before they reach the shops, and the more fragile the fruit or vegetables (lettuce or berries), the more they are sprayed in a bid to increase their shelf life.

When eating organic vegetables like carrots it is better not to peel but just scrub the skins, as much of their nutrient value is just under the skin. But if you are using non-organic fruit and vegetables, it is wise to peel them before eating or cooking them. Discard the outer leaves of cabbages and other green vegetables. Washing can't alter the pesticides absorbed in the fruit or vegetables, but peeling can lower the residues by about three quarters. Try to eat a wide variety of fruits and vegetables as specific pesticides are used for specific crops and if you keep changing your choices, you should avoid eating too much of a given pesticide.

YOUR HOME

Your home could harbour higher levels of toxins than outside because you are exposed to them more frequently and you are also in closer contact with them. So think about the cleaning products you use indoors and be aware of the air freshener or sprays you breathe in repeatedly or the washing powder that leaves residues near your skin.

Most air fresheners work by using nerve-deadening agents to stop you detecting smells or by putting chemical fragrances into the air. You can now buy natural air fresheners, or you could burn essential oils to give a lovely fragrance.

You can also clear the air with houseplants. They absorb the carbon dioxide we exhale and release the oxygen that is vital for us to breathe. Some plants, such as the spider plant, also remove some air pollutants.

Consider changing to more natural choices that aren't so heavily laden with chemicals. As with skincare products, 'natural' cleaning and domestic products are increasingly available even in ordinary super-markets. Read the labels carefully and go for those with the fewest

AVOIDING PLASTICS

Here are some tips for reducing the amount of plastic you use:

- Don't wrap food in cling film; use greaseproof paper instead.
- Don't store fatty food in cling film as the chemicals will leach into foods with a high-fat content. Instead store in a glass dish with a glass lid – and if you must use cling film in place of a glass lid, make sure the food does not touch the plastic.
- If you do use cling film, choose one made of low-density polyethylene (LDPE) and not PVC which can transfer EDCs from the plastic to the food.
- Avoid food that needs to be microwaved in a plastic container.
- Use glass bottles instead of plastic where possible.
- If you use a plastic bottle choose one that states it is BPA free.
- Don't refill old ordinary plastic bottles; the older the bottle and the more damaged it gets the greater the risk of BPA leaching into the water.
- Don't leave plastic water bottles sitting in direct sunlight as heat increases the leaching effect of the chemicals.
- Don't rinse out plastic bottles or containers in very hot water as BPA leaches out fifty-five times faster than normal.
- Be careful also of takeaway hot drinks in plastic cups because chemicals will leach out quickly from the plastic.
- Reduce the amount of tinned foods and drinks you have because of the plastic coating inside the cans.

chemicals. There is a range of natural products at www.naturalhealth practice.com.

Another option is to revert to simple old-fashioned methods such as cleaning windows with vinegar and water. Use natural wax for furniture polish and, to freshen your carpets, try sprinkling them with baking soda, scented with two drops of lavender essential oil, and leave for fifteen minutes before vacuuming.

It is particularly advisable to avoid pesticides (in the garden, to protect your pets from fleas or to rid your house of insects or rodents) as studies show they can disrupt the female hormone system.[11]

Nobody really knows what the long-term effects are of all these chemicals on your health, but I believe, if you are trying to deal with PCOS, it is worthwhile detoxifying your environment where possible. If you have to expose yourself to chemicals (buying a hot drink from a café in a plastic cup, for example), don't worry, it's not the end of the world. What really counts is the fact that you do whatever you can to reduce your chemical exposure the majority of the time.

PART THREE

LIVING WITH PCOS

CHAPTER 11

YOUR FERTILITY

By following all the advice I have given so far in this book, you should be well on your way to managing your PCOS, and – with time and patience – there's every chance you may be able to reverse it. It would be wrong to expect instant results, but you may already be noticing improvements in your weight, your skin, your hair and your general health. If you're lucky, you might even start to ovulate once more, because possibly one of the most important changes my natural approaches can make is to help your body establish a normal, regular menstrual cycle.

You may know that PCOS is, very sadly, one of the leading causes of infertility. Unless you ovulate, you simply won't be able to conceive naturally. If you can get your hormones back in balance, however, and your ovaries working properly, your chances of conception will dramatically improve. (And if things don't happen naturally, be reassured that fertility treatment has good success rates, even if you have PCOS; but it has an even better chance if you follow my guidelines and get the condition under control.)

If you want to get pregnant, you just need a clear of plan of action so that you know what you should be doing and when.

FOR THE UNDER-THIRTY-FIVES

If you are in your twenties and early thirties you are lucky – you have time on your side. I suggest you follow my nutritional recommendations for six months, without medication, to see if you do start to ovulate and conceive naturally. Trust me – it can work.

Obviously, you'll need to come off the Pill (otherwise you'll have no way of knowing whether my plan is working) and, when you are actively trying to conceive, stop taking any herbs and just take vitamins, minerals and Omega 3 fats.

If you have been prescribed the insulin sensitizer drug metformin, it's a good idea to reread Chapter 5 and make sure you're not inadvertently taking any of the nutrients that contraindicate using this drug.

To boost your chances even further, it's worth asking your partner to read this chapter and follow the fertility recommendations himself to make sure his sperm health is as good as it can possibly be.

FOR THE OVER-THIRTY-FIVES

Once you get to your mid-thirties, your fertility – even if you don't have PCOS – will be starting gradually to decline. If you have PCOS and want to get pregnant, you don't have time to hang around.

It is worth seeking advice from your doctor, and making sure you know exactly what infertility treatment is available to you. You may not need it, but at least you will have a plan of action, and the wheels of infertility treatment can be set in motion, without wasting any precious time.

If you are already taking fertility drugs, such as clomiphene (see page 174), there is absolutely no problem with you following my natural approach simultaneously. In fact, it's the most sensible thing you could do, but don't take the herbs, just use my dietary recommendations and the supplements (see Chapters 4 and 5).

Don't embark on any fertility treatment alone until your partner has been fully investigated. If it turns out that both of you need a fertility boost – either nutritionally or medically – it's far better for you to start at the same time. You should know that up to 30 per cent of fertility problems can be attributed to the man, so your PCOS might not be the issue at all.

Although the under-thirty-fives normally find it much easier to get pregnant, if you have PCOS, you may find it easier to get pregnant as you get older. This is because it is possible that your PCOS may improve with age. As we get older the number of follicles in our ovaries reduce and in most cases, this makes getting pregnant harder. But if you have PCOS, fewer follicles can be helpful because normally the problem with PCOS is having too many follicles.

Research has shown that by the age of thirty-five, women who have PCOS will have had as many successful pregnancies as those who don't, even without having fertility treatment.[1] Some experts believe that with PCOS, the ovaries age more slowly, giving you an extra two years of reproductive life over someone who doesn't have the condition.[2]

I cannot stress how vital the diet and lifestyle recommendations are in helping you to get pregnant.[3] Follow the advice in Chapters 4 and 5 and complement it with the recommendations in this chapter.

BOOST YOUR FERTILITY

Here's how to give yourself the best possible chance of getting pregnant:

1. EAT WELL

It couldn't be more important for you to follow all the dietary advice in Chapter 4. This will not only give you control over your PCOS, but all the antioxidants, fibre, essential fats, good-quality protein and carbohydrates contained in the recommended foods really will give you the best chance of conceiving naturally and will significantly boost the success rate of any fertility treatment.

Here's a brief reminder of my seven dietary steps:

1. Switch to unrefined carbohydrates and never go more than three hours without food to balance blood-sugar levels (see page 42).
2. Eat oily fish and foods rich in Omega 3s (nuts, seeds and oils) to help your body to become more sensitive to insulin so it can overcome insulin resistance (see page 49).
3. Cut back on dairy products to control levels of male hormones (see page 50).
4. Eat more vegetables and pulses (organic, if possible) (see page 55).
5. Cut back on alcohol and avoid sugar and artificial sweeteners (see page 56).
6. Cut down on caffeine to support your adrenal glands (see page 58).
7. Cut down on saturated fats and eliminate trans fats to get more control over the potentially damaging inflammatory processes PCOS causes in the body (see page 60).

It is important to stop or cut down on alcohol, which makes it more difficult to get pregnant[4] and that applies to both you *and* your partner. Alcohol can lower sperm counts and will also block the body's ability to absorb fertility-boosting nutrients like zinc. It can also cause abnormalities in the head of the sperm which is important for healthy fertilization.[5]

It is also well worth cutting back on caffeine: four cups of coffee (or any caffeinated drink) a day have been shown to make it 26 per cent less likely that you will conceive,[6] and drinking only two cups of coffee (200mg caffeine) a day is associated with a 25 per cent increased risk of miscarriage.[7] And get your partner to switch to decaffeinated too. Problems with sperm health are connected with increased coffee intake.[8]

Studies also show that increasing your intake of healthy fats (and cutting back on unhealthy trans fats) will increase your chance of ovulating.[9] Adding vegetable protein (tofu, pulses, nuts) to each meal to keep your blood sugar in balance also seems to boost your chances of ovulating.[10]

2. LIVE WELL

If you really do want to get pregnant, you need to follow my other guidelines in terms of reducing stress, exercising, sleeping well, and cutting back on your toxic overload. This applies to you *and* your partner.

If you smoke, stop. You are twice as likely to get pregnant if you don't smoke,[11] and smoking is linked to 5,000 miscarriages per year.[12] The chemicals in tobacco smoke can damage DNA in sperm, making it harder to conceive and increasing the risk of a miscarriage (nature will always work on survival of the fittest). Smoking can also affect the sperm count, motility and the morphology (the shape of the sperm), having a negative effect on the head of the sperm, making it harder to fertilize an egg.[13]

You should also know that smoking will reduce your chances of success at infertility treatment. If couples smoke during the IVF cycle, the number of eggs retrieved is decreased by 40 per cent and the success rate drops (44 per cent for non-smokers and 24 per cent for smokers).[14]

It is worth asking your partner to avoid hot baths, tight underpants, sitting for long periods and using a laptop on his lap as these can reduce sperm health too.[15]

If you are doing everything you can to control your PCOS, you certainly won't want other factors which can stop you conceiving to get in the way. A combination of four negative lifestyle factors (such as drinking tea or coffee, smoking and consuming alcohol) can make it take seven times longer for a couple to get pregnant.[16]

I know making these changes will require effort and commitment from you and your partner but it really is *very* important that you do this. And it's not just me who thinks so. Research scientists universally agree that lifestyle modification *can* assist couples to conceive spontaneously or optimize their chances of conception with assisted reproductive technology.[17]

3. TAKE SUPPLEMENTS

The PCOS supplements (see Chapter 5) you take will help to regulate your cycle, improve ovulation and boost your fertility generally. However, when you are actively trying to conceive you need to take a multivitamin and mineral designed for fertility and also a separate vitamin C and the same fish oil you were taking before. Research by the US Harvard School of Public Health showed that regular use of multivitamin supplements can decrease the risk of ovulatory infertility.[18]

I have outlined below a recommended supplement programme containing the most important supplements if you are trying to conceive, and have then given details about each one. They are mostly all contained in your fertility multivitamin and mineral for you and your partner, apart from the vitamin C and Omega 3 fish oils.

Your fertility supplement programme at a glance
- Good multivitamin and mineral designed for fertility – containing folic acid, zinc, selenium, vitamin E, the amino acids L-arginine and L-carnitine (in addition for the man) and vitamin D. (I recommend NHP's Fertility Support for Women and Fertility Support for Men available from health food shops or www.naturalhealthpractice.com.)
- Vitamin C
- Omega 3 fish oils

Folic acid

All women, whether or not they have PCOS, should start to take folic acid when they decide to try to conceive. This can prevent spina bifida (a birth defect in which the backbone and spinal canal do not close before birth) and is part of the essential B-complex family of vitamins that are necessary to produce the genetic materials DNA and RNA. Together with vitamin B12, folic acid works to ensure that your baby's genetic codes are intact.

Take: 400μg of folic acid daily as part of your fertility multivitamin and mineral.

Zinc

Zinc is an essential component of genetic material. A zinc deficiency can cause chromosome changes in either men or women, leading to reduced fertility and an increased risk of miscarriage. Zinc is found in high concentrations in the sperm and is needed to make the outer layer and tail of the sperm; it is, therefore, essential for sperm health. To show you how powerful these nutrients are, in one study men who were subfertile showed a 74 per cent increase in total sperm count after taking a combination of zinc and folic acid.[19]

Take: 30mg of zinc daily as part of your fertility multivitamin and mineral.

Selenium

Selenium is an antioxidant that helps to protect your body from highly reactive chemical fragments called free radicals. For this reason, selenium can prevent chromosome breakage, which is known to be a cause of birth defects and miscarriages. Good levels of selenium are also essential to maximize sperm formation and selenium supplements have been found to increase sperm count, motility and the number of normal sperm in infertile men.[20]

Take: 100μg of selenium daily as part of your fertility multivitamin and mineral.

Vitamin E

Vitamin E is another powerful antioxidant and has been shown to increase fertility when given to both men and women. In men, vitamin E helps to increase fertilization rates during ICSI (intracytoplasmic sperm injection – see page 180).[21] Taken with vitamin C, it is particularly useful for woman over thirty-five as these antioxidants have been shown to significantly reduce age-related ovulation decline.[22]

Take: 200mg of vitamin E daily as part of your fertility multivitamin and mineral.

Vitamin D

Vitamin D is also active in reducing your insulin resistance and inflammation, but it can assist in balancing your immune system too, which is very important for pregnancy. Vitamin D, like the Omega 3 fats, does a great job of lowering the Th1 autoimmune response, but it also helps to promote the Th2 cells your body needs to maintain a pregnancy.[23, 24]

Vitamin D is also involved in male fertility as it contributes to increasing sperm motility and improving the number of normally formed sperm.[25]

Given the widespread deficiencies it is a good idea to get tested for vitamin D and then supplement to correct the deficiency and then retest after three months (go to www.naturalhealthpractice.com for a simple finger-prick home test).

Take: At least 2.5µg of vitamin D daily as part of your fertility multivitamin and mineral.

Amino acids

Two amino acids, L-arginine and L-carnitine, are particularly important for male fertility: L-arginine is essential for healthy sperm production and protects the sperm against oxidative damage;[26] and the higher the levels of L-carnitine in sperm cells, the higher the sperm count and motility.[27]

Take: 300mg of L-arginine and 100mg of L-carnitine daily as part of your fertility multivitamin and mineral.

Vitamin C

Vitamin C, another antioxidant, is beneficial for women who appear to be resistant to the fertility drug clomiphene (see page 174).[28] It has also been shown to increase pregnancy rates in women going through IVF treatment and can boost sperm counts in men by up to a third.[29, 30]

Antioxidants in general (and that includes zinc, selenium, vitamin C and vitamin E) have been shown to have a major impact on male fertility. A review of thirty-four studies with men going for IVF/ICSI cycles has shown that when men take antioxidants their partner is five times more likely to have a live birth compared to those who did not take the antioxidants.[31]

Take: 500mg of vitamin C twice daily.

Omega 3 fats

These essential fatty acids that we get from oily fish, nuts and seeds have far-reaching effects for your fertility.

I recommend women with PCOS take Omega 3 supplements to help control their insulin resistance and to reduce the inflammation that results from the body's overactive immune system (which is trying to deal with all the insulin washing around in the blood). But if the oils calm your immune system, this can also help you get and stay pregnant. So the theory is that in order for your body to stay pregnant, your immune system has to quieten down, so it doesn't register a baby (whose DNA is only half yours) as an invader. Normally, if your body detects something foreign it will try to expel it from the body. This can be another reason why women with uncontrolled PCOS find it so hard to get or stay pregnant.

In one study, twenty-two women with high levels of the blood-clotting antibodies shown to cause recurrent miscarriages were given fish oil, resulting in pregnancies in all twenty-two women – one woman had twins.[32]

Your immune system also produces natural killer cells (NK cells). They sound frightening, but they are useful when deployed to control rapidly dividing cells like cancer. Some (but certainly not all) medics believe that some women have higher levels of NK cells which attack a developing foetus as the cells grow and divide. But research shows that fish oil, specifically EPA which is high in fish oils, decreases NK killer cell activity by 48 per cent. It was interesting to note that the other oils tested – linseed, GLA (e.g. evening primrose oil) and DHA did not cause any change in NK activity.[33] The dose of EPA used for the trial was 720mg, so choose a supplement containing over 700mg in two capsules.

Fish oils can help fertility in other ways. Experts believe one reason for miscarriage and infertility could be an imbalance in the immune system which makes the auto-immune response (called Th1) dominate over what is called the suppressive response (Th2).[34] Studies show that recurrent implantation failure with IVF can be associated with a predominantly Th1 response.[35] The conventional treatment for this is powerful drugs (anti-TNF-alpha drug or IVIg), but research into fish oil has shown that it can inhibit TNF alpha by as much as 90 per cent, making it as effective as the drug.[36]

Omega 3 fats are also important for your partner because semen is rich in prostaglandins, which are produced from these Omega 3 fats. Men with inadequate levels of these beneficial prostaglandins can have poor sperm quality, abnormal sperm, poor motility or low count,[37] but studies show that sperm count can be increased significantly by taking Omega 3 fish oil supplements to up the levels of prostaglandins.[38]

Take: 770mg EPA and 510mg DHA fish oils daily.

HOW DO I KNOW IF I AM OVULATING?

It is possible to still have periods but not be ovulating, so even though your periods may be fairly regular, I'm afraid you can't assume you are ovulating every month. But there are ways to check:

Ultrasound scan

Ask your doctor for an ultrasound scan, which is the most conclusive way to know whether or not you are ovulating (see pages 28–9). If you have difficulty getting one done, then contact my clinic and we can arrange for a referral during the nutritional consultation. (See Useful Resources, page 217.)

Ovulation kits

Readily available from pharmacies or online, these kits work by registering the surge in luteinizing hormone (LH – see page 14) that occurs two to three days before ovulation. But if you have PCOS you are likely to have continually high levels of LH, so regardless of which day you do the test, the sample will register as positive. Unfortunately, this is a false positive.

The only way you can be sure the kit is working is if you manage to get very low LH readings on some days in the month. This would mean a high LH reading could indicate ovulation in your case. When you follow my diet and lifestyle suggestions you might start to see this happening.

Cervical mucus

The best way to self-test whether or not you are ovulating is to learn to identify the mucus produced by the glands lining your cervical canal which changes consistency just before ovulation. Normal mucus is thick and sticky, hostile to sperm (acidic) and forms a plug over the cervix, but a few days before ovulation, it should become watery, stretchy and clear, making your vagina alkaline and providing nourishment and swimming canals for sperm. Once ovulation has taken place, the mucus becomes hostile once more.

To test the mucus, blot yourself with white toilet paper when you are on the toilet. You may see mucus on the paper, in which case, lightly apply a finger to it, then pull gently away to test its ability to stretch. If it feels slippery like raw egg white and can stretch between your first finger and thumb up to several inches before breaking, it is fertile; if it is dry, thick and sticky, it is the more acid, infertile mucus. As it changes to become fertile, this is a sign that ovulation is about to take place.

Body temperature

In most women, their temperature rises a few degrees after ovulation and stays higher until menstruation, so they can test for ovulation by keeping a record of this (taking a reading first thing in the morning before getting out of bed each day).

If you have PCOS though, and no regular cycle, you would need to take your temperature for many months before you'd notice a pattern emerging. Moreover, many factors can affect your temperature such as alcohol, exercise, stress, anxiety, fever, drugs and shift work, so unfortunately, body temperature is not an accurate test for ovulation when you have PCOS. I would suggest you concentrate on measuring cervical mucus changes instead as this can be checked very easily when you go to the toilet.

Other fertility signs
- Position of the cervix: prior to ovulation, the cervix moves higher in the vaginal canal and becomes softer and opens.

- Ovulation pain: some women can *feel* that they are ovulating as they experience a sharp pain or ache.
- Spotting: a small loss of blood may occur around ovulation (any more blood loss, other than a period, should be checked with your doctor).
- Tender breasts: in some women their breasts become tender after ovulation.

3. WATCH YOUR WEIGHT

Not only will losing weight ease your PCOS symptoms, but studies show that if you are a healthy weight, you will get pregnant more quickly, and if you do decide to have IVF, your chance of success will be higher. Even a small 5–10 per cent loss in weight can have a remarkable effect on your ovaries,[39, 40] and slimming down also protects you, to some extent, against the miscarriage risk so commonly associated with PCOS.[41]

Weight loss also (if you are overweight) increases effectiveness of the drugs used to stimulate ovulation. In fact, many IVF clinics will not treat overweight women who have a BMI (body mass index – see page 86) of above 30 because obesity has such a negative impact on success rates. Your man should watch his weight too, as there is an increased risk of infertility or poor sperm quality and quantity in men who are overweight or obese.[42]

4. CONSIDER OTHER NATURAL THERAPIES

You may want to combine your diet and lifestyle changes with a few sessions of acupuncture, homeopathy, reflexology, hypnotherapy, aromatherapy or cranial osteopathy. These natural therapies can be beneficial for managing your PCOS and will, in most cases, enhance the effect of the other changes you are making in your life. There is even some evidence that they can help boost your fertility.

Choose the therapy which appeals to you the most – perhaps counselling or hypnotherapy for dealing with the stress and emotional upheaval of getting pregnant, or acupuncture, reflexology or homeopathy to get your hormones back in balance.

Acupuncture

Acupuncture is believed to help balance hormones, kick-start or regulate the cycle, increase ovulation, reduce stress and improve blood flow to the womb, which can aid in successful implantation and improve the success rate of an IVF treatment.

In one study, acupuncture was found to have helped 38 per cent of women with PCOS either to have regular ovulation or become pregnant.[43] During an IVF cycle, acupuncture has shown to help the success of that cycle.[44] And some studies show that acupuncture may also be useful for your partner as it can increase the number of normal sperm, so consider going for a session together.[45]

Homeopathy

Homeopathy has been shown to help with infertility in both men[46] and women.[47] A number of homeopathic remedies are used, including pulsatilla, argentums nitricum, selenenium metallicum and lycopodium, but I always recommend an individual consultation (which looks not only at PCOS, but also your likes and dislikes, moods and family history), so you can be sure the remedies are right for you.

Reflexology

Reflexology aims to stimulate reflex points on the feet which are linked to the meridians connected to certain organs. It can also help with stress reduction.

There haven't been many studies associating reflexology with PCOS, but it is believed to be beneficial. In one small trial in Denmark, nineteen out of sixty-one women, who were aged over thirty and had been trying to conceive for nearly seven years, conceived within six months of completing the treatment.[48]

Hypnotherapy

Hypnotherapy can be useful if you are fearful of being pregnant. The mind can exert powerful influence over the body, and if part of you has doubts about being a mother, coping with a baby or how it might affect your relationship with your partner, hypnotherapy can give you some clarity on whether this is really what you want.

Infertility could be making you stressed and anxious, and the fear of not getting pregnant could be worsening the stress which, in turn, can be affecting ovulation and conception. Hypnotherapy could be useful with this.[49] Studies show that this approach can be of value if hormonal imbalance is causing infertility problems (which is very much the case with PCOS),[50] and also during IVF treatment. In one study, a group of couples that had hypnotherapy had a clinical pregnancy rate of 53.1 per cent compared to a rate of 30.2 per cent for the group that had not. The results suggest that hypnosis during IVF can help to increase implantation and pregnancy rate.[51]

Aromatherapy

Although there has been no research into the effectiveness of aromatherapy in either PCOS or fertility, it has been shown to help with stress and anxiety, both of which are factors associated with PCOS.[52]

Aromatherapy uses specific essential oils to regulate hormones and relieve stress. A number of oils are often used for fertility including lavender, clary sage, geranium, jasmine, melissa, rose, sandalwood, neroli and ylang ylang.

Cranial osteopathy

Cranial osteopaths use their hands to sense subtle rhythmical changes in the skull to diagnose stresses in the body and release congestion and restriction. This can boost blood flow to the womb and relieve any congestion around the pelvic area and reproductive organs.

GETTING MEDICAL HELP

If you have been battling with PCOS for some time, and you're not conceiving as quickly as you'd like, do tell your doctor you are hoping to get pregnant. There are various tests available which can eliminate the possibility of other problems which might be contributing to your infertility.

FERTILITY TESTS

Although you may already have been tested for PCOS (which is most likely to be to blame for your infertility), you should also rule out any other problems that may be affecting your ability to conceive.

Blocked fallopian tubes

Blocked fallopian tubes can account for 20 per cent of female infertility. They could be something you were born with, or can be caused by infection, pelvic inflammatory disease or scar tissue from any previous surgery.

You should find out if your tubes are blocked because, if they are, you may be moved swiftly to the IVF stage of infertility treatment, bypassing the earlier, more time-consuming stages. If your GP decides your tubes should be checked, you may be offered one of three different procedures:

- A hysterosalpingogram (HSG) – you will be X-rayed as a dye is passed through the fallopian tubes.
- An HyCoSy (hystero-contrast sonography) – this is where a special fluid is injected into the womb (via the cervix) and its progress monitored via ultrasound (the monitor is inserted into the vagina).

- A laparoscopy – this is where a tiny camera is inserted through a small cut in the belly button (under general anaesthetic) to check the condition of your tubes.

In my opinion the HyCoSy is the better choice for checking fallopian-tube patency (as it is called medically) as it avoids the use of both X-rays and a general anaesthetic.

Semen analysis

Your partner should have a semen analysis. If sperm count is low you may be offered ICSI (see page 180), but getting him to take on board my nutritional changes could be enough to see great improvements.

ASSISTED REPRODUCTION

This includes all forms of medical help from drugs (like clomiphene) to full IVF.

If your main focus right now is getting pregnant, and you are aged thirty-five or older, I would recommend you ignore or reject the various drugs and surgical procedures that are available to ease your PCOS symptoms, and instead concentrate specifically on your fertility.

There is an established and accepted series of treatments and interventions designed specifically to help women with PCOS get pregnant.[53] The treatment falls into three sequential stages, one following the other, each progressively invasive (and more expensive). You are unlikely to be moved on to each stage until it is clear that the previous stage has not worked.

Before you embark on any medical treatment, your GP or gynaecologist will be expected to talk to you about the importance of diet, exercise, stress reduction, stopping smoking and reducing alcohol consumption. So if you've already been working through this book, you should have a head start here. But when the medical profession agrees with nutritionists that diet and lifestyle are important in the quest to get pregnant, you can be absolutely sure that these steps are crucial.

First-line treatment: ovulation

Unless you are prepared to accept a donor egg, you cannot get pregnant unless you ovulate, so the first line of attack is to boost your ovulation, with a drug called clomiphene citrate. Clomiphene is available on the NHS and it is the main drug given for PCOS and when a woman is not ovulating. It is an anti-oestrogenic drug which is taken on days two to five of your cycle. If you are not having a cycle, you would be given another drug to induce a bleed and then the clomiphene is started on day two of the bleed.

Clomiphene works by making your brain think there is not enough oestrogen in your blood, so it encourages your pituitary gland to increase the level of FSH (follicle-stimulating hormone), which prompts the follicles in the ovaries to – ideally – produce an egg. When the clomiphene is stopped on day five, the brain records a return to a relatively high amount of oestrogen and triggers a surge of LH (luteinizing hormone), which causes the egg to be released from the ovary.

Clomiphene has a good success rate – 75 to 80 per cent of women taking it ovulate and 29 per cent subsequently have a baby.[54] Seventy-five per cent of pregnancies are achieved during the first three cycles of treatment.[55]

If clomiphene hasn't worked after six cycles, it is probably not going to work for you and it may be time to try something else. In any case, your doctor is unlikely to recommend you take it for more than six ovulatory cycles as there could be an increased risk of ovarian cancer if it is taken for longer.[56] Clomiphene can be very effective, but it can also increase the risk of womb cancer when taken for any length of time[57] and common side effects can include headaches, depression, fatigue and hot flushes (because it is an anti-oestrogen). There is a

10 per cent risk of a multiple pregnancy (twins or triplets), because clomiphene increases the number of follicles. Also, because it is an anti-oestrogen, there are women who experience changes in cervical mucus (more acid, so more hostile to sperm – see page 167) and the womb lining (which becomes thinner), making implantation more difficult which can increase the miscarriage rate. So ironically, it may be helping you to conceive, but making it harder to stay pregnant.

With clomiphene, you are most likely to be started on the lowest dose of 50mg per day, but this might be raised to a maximum of 150mg per day. Studies show that doses higher than 150mg do not improve the drug's effectiveness in women with PCOS.

Some women, particularly those with PCOS, can turn out to be clomiphene resistant. This is more likely to be the case if you are obese, insulin resistant and also have higher levels of male hormones.[58]

You will need to be monitored with an ultrasound scan while taking clompihene, at least on the first cycle or longer, if possible, in case it doesn't work straight away or doesn't work at all for you and you are not ovulating while taking it. Scanning will show clearly if the dose needs adjusting because your doctor will be able to see how your ovaries are responding to the drug. The doctor will also check whether you are producing too many follicles (you might be told not to try to conceive that month due to the risk of a large multiple pregnancy) and the dose can be altered. The ultrasound scan can also show whether the drug is thinning your womb lining (so making miscarriage more likely).

Sometimes another drug called human chorionic gonadotrophin (hCG) is given in the middle of the cycle while you are taking clomiphene. This drug makes your ovary release its dominant (biggest) follicle. It is given by injection and has to be timed exactly. If given too soon, it may actually stop ovulation and can increase the risk of a multiple pregnancy and ovarian hyperstimulation syndrome (OHSS – see page 180). But the research shows it does *not* increase your chances of getting pregnant if you have PCOS.[59]

Some research has also indicated combining clomiphene with metformin (see page 34) to increase your chances of getting pregnant, but this is not widely recommended.[60] It is suggested that metformin used in PCOS should only be given to women with glucose intolerance or Type 2 diabetes (not just insulin resistance) and should not be used routinely for ovulation induction.

The Royal College of Obstetricians and Gynaecologists has published a book called *Current Management of PCOS* that concludes that metformin is overused in the treatment of PCOS and is ineffective either on its own or in combination to treat infertility, to achieve a pregnancy or to prevent miscarriage.[61]

Other drugs that might be used to help women with PCOS include tamoxifen (which, like clomiphene is an anti-oestrogen) and also aromatase inhibitors (like letrozole). They can be as effective as clomiphene at stimulating ovulation, but are not licensed to be used for fertility.[62]

If you choose to take clomiphene, make sure you are taking vitamin C supplements because they can be helpful in overcoming clomiphene resistance. The amino acid N-acetyl cysteine has also been used alongside clomiphene in women with PCOS who are clomiphene resistant. In one study, the combination of clomiphene with N-acetyl cysteine increased both ovulation and pregnancy rates by 49.3 per cent compared to only 21.3 per cent when clomiphene was taken alone.[63]

I do not normally recommend taking herbs like black cohosh when taking medication that can affect your hormones because they can have a powerful effect and may clash with the medication, but one study has shown that black cohosh can improve the effectiveness of clomiphene, helping with better womb thickness and higher progesterone levels and resulting in higher pregnancy rates. It might, therefore, be worth trying black cohosh with your medication on days one to twelve *only* of your cycle.[64]

Second-line treatment

If the first-line drug treatment does not work, your GP or gynaecologist is likely to recommend using FSH (follicle-stimulating hormone) or perhaps suggest surgery.

FSH: The aim with this next step is to increase your FSH levels: just enough to make a number of follicles on the ovary grow in order to produce one mature egg, but not so much that you could end up with a multiple pregnancy. Moving on to FSH from clomiphene results in a 72 per cent chance of having a baby,[65] but this step does need commitment, as you have to give yourself daily injections and be monitored carefully by your doctor so that you are only developing one egg.

These days, most specialists start with the lowest possible dose and observe your ovaries by ultrasound, gradually increasing the dose until follicles start to develop and maintaining the dose at that point. Your doctor would decide how often you need to be examined and when to vary the dose. The other approach is to start on a higher dose of FSH and reduce it as soon as your follicles show signs of development.

Research suggests that the first protocol is safest,[66] and as starting at a higher dose requires more monitoring and expertise to get it right and both protocols achieve the same success rates, it seems more logical to start on the lower dose and work up.

Surgery – ovarian drilling: Although it sounds rather dramatic, this surgical procedure is frequently carried out on women with PCOS and has been shown to make ovulation more likely, particularly if you are resistant to the ovary-stimulating drug clomiphene.

Under a general anaesthetic, the surgeon inserts cameras and tubes through tiny (laparoscopic) holes in your abdomen, and one or both ovaries are 'drilled' to destroy the inner ovarian tissue that produces testosterone, leaving the delicate surface of the ovary intact. The procedure comes with all the usual risks of surgery, and there is an additional concern that it could destroy the ovaries completely, causing ovarian failure and infertility, but it has been shown to trigger ovulation in 80 per cent of women with PCOS and result in a 50 per cent pregnancy rate.[67] It also makes the ovaries more responsive to clomiphene.

Ovarian drilling is thought to be of particular benefit for women with high LH levels or low body weight, and is considered a better option for them than clomiphene. This is because clomiphene is an anti-oestrogen; if you have PCOS and are slim, it can make the lining of your womb too thin (increasing the likelihood of miscarriage) or even dry up the cervical mucus, making the environment hostile to sperm, so that they are unable to swim to reach the egg and they die off.

Research shows that ovarian drilling is as successful as clomiphene for stimulating ovulation in women with PCOS,[68] and as successful as using FSH.[69]

Unfortunately, half of all women who have ovarian drilling do not ovulate after the surgery. In such cases, another course of clomiphene can be given after three months, and if ovulation still has not occurred after six months, FSH is very often added to the mix as well.

If you do decide to have ovarian drilling, I recommend taking supplements of the amino acid N-acetyl cysteine (see page 76) as this can significantly improve ovulation rates, pregnancy rates and live birth rates, as well as reducing the risk of miscarriage.[70]

Third-line treatment

If the first- and second-line treatments are unsuccessful, you will normally be recommended for IVF.

However, with PCOS, as the main issue in helping you to get pregnant is triggering ovulation, I would suggest that you try a couple of cycles of IUI (intrauterine insemination) before embarking on IVF. This is a procedure which involves washing and preparing a sample of your partner's sperm and inserting it directly into your womb, ready to fertilize an egg (after your ovaries have been stimulated to produce one). It is less costly and less invasive than full IVF, so as long as you know that your fallopian tubes are clear and your partner's semen analysis is good, you have little to lose by having a couple of IUI cycles.

There are a number of reasons why IUI has an advantage over natural conception when you have PCOS:

- Inserting the sperm directly into your womb through a catheter shortens the distance between the egg and the sperm.
- It bypasses any problem you might have with cervical mucus which may be too thick or too acidic (known as hostile mucus) to allow the sperm through.
- Your partner's sperm is washed and prepared before inserting to optimize its survival and fertilization chances.
- Sperm is only inserted if ovulation occurs and at exactly the right point (as detected by ultrasound scan) in the ovulation cycle to maximize the likelihood that it will work.

You would need to be monitored carefully through the IUI to avoid the risk of multiple pregnancies from the ovulation stimulation. Success rates are around 10 to 15 per cent, depending on your age. Naturally, I recommend you get your diet and lifestyle in place before you start IUI to give it the best chance of working.

IVF (in-vitro fertilization): This is an assisted-conception procedure whereby eggs are removed from your ovaries and fertilized with your partner's sperm outside your body, then put back into the womb as embryos. In the UK, there is a rule permitting only two embryos to be transferred into the womb when a woman is aged under forty and no more than three if she is over forty.

You will be given fertility drugs to stimulate ovulation and the drugs used and the dosages depend on the individual fertility clinics. However, when you have PCOS, there is an increased chance that these drugs could cause you to produce too many eggs, putting you at risk of a more serious problem called OHSS (ovarian hyperstimulation syndrome), where the large amount of follicles stimulated during IVF cause a shift of fluid and protein balance in the body. This makes the ovaries become enlarged and fluid can build up in the abdomen.

Different clinics use different combinations of drugs, but specific protocols have been published in the medical literature in relation to women with PCOS having IVF and the standard one mentioned in the PCOS consensus statement is a long protocol with FSH.[71]

Throughout this highly technical process, you can still help yourself nutritionally and all the dietary recommendations mentioned in this book still apply while you're undergoing IVF. Also, as the problem with OHSS is a change in fluid and protein in the body, make sure you have plenty of water and herb teas and increase your intake of good-quality protein as you go through the IVF cycle (including eggs, fish, nuts and seeds). Some IVF clinics suggest you increase protein and fluids by drinking large amounts of milk, but I would not recommend this approach, particularly if you have PCOS, as you may be vulnerable to the higher amounts of hormones in the dairy products (see pages 50–51). Stick to water, herb teas and fish, nuts and seeds instead.

It is also thought that taking metformin during the IVF cycle may decrease the risk of OHSS in women with PCOS as it seems to stop the ovaries from becoming overstimulated.[72] And taking metformin during an IVF cycle may also help to improve fertilization rates in women with PCOS and also pregnancy rates.[73]

ICSI (intracytoplasmic sperm injection): If your partner has problems with his sperm (low count or high abnormal forms), you may be offered an ICSI treatment rather than IVF.

The drug procedure will be exactly the same for you, but with ICSI the sperm is injected directly into the egg (instead of your egg and your partner's sperm being put in the dish together for fertilization).

IVM (in-vitro maturation): This is a fairly new technique, but it seems to be particularly good for women with PCOS and those for whom there is a risk of OHSS.

Instead of retrieving mature eggs triggered by drug stimulation, immature eggs are retrieved from the ovaries, then matured in a dish with LH and FSH over twenty-four hours, after which they are fertilized using the ICSI technique of injecting the sperm into the egg. This process does away with the need for daily drugs and allows multiple immature eggs to be collected.

At the time of writing, about 400 babies worldwide have been born using IVM. The HFEA (Human Fertilization and Embryology Authority) in the UK lists the clinics that offer this technique (see www.hfea.gov.uk/fertility-treatment-options-in-vitro-maturation).

MISCARRIAGE

Unfortunately, women with PCOS are three times more likely to miscarry. This is thought to be due to typically higher LH levels which can affect the quality of the eggs causing a miscarriage.[74]

It really is so important that you put in place all the dietary and supplement recommendations in Chapters 4 and 5 because these can be instrumental in reducing the risk of miscarriage by getting your hormones back in balance and improving the quality of your eggs.

Some research is beginning to suggest that metformin may help to prevent early miscarriage for women with PCOS,[75] but there does not seem to be any advantage in continuing with it after the first trimester.[76] This will be covered in more detail in the next chapter.

TRYING TO CONCEIVE

If you have PCOS and you want to get pregnant, I cannot stress strongly enough just how vital it is for you to put in place my lifestyle and nutritional recommendations. These changes to your diet and the addition of specific supplements and herbs really will increase your chances of conceiving, staying pregnant and having a happy, healthy baby.

In many cases, these measures will be enough to get your body back on track, triggering ovulation, so that you will conceive naturally. But if you do need medical help, your chances of success are massively improved if you're eating the right foods and supplements, exercising, watching your weight and avoiding tobacco and alcohol.[77]

For many of you this will mean making tough choices and some challenging lifestyle changes, but my methods work. If you really do want to get pregnant, it's got to be worth it.

CHAPTER 12

PREGNANCY

I sincerely hope you will use the natural solutions from this book to help you get pregnant, or at least use them alongside IVF if you have to go down that road.

With luck, you will be successful. I sincerely hope so. And when you do conceive, you mustn't slip back into poor eating habits. Keep my dietary recommendations and certain supplements going right through your pregnancy. It may be tempting to think that once you are pregnant you have achieved your aim and can do what you want, but the food you eat and the way you look after yourself when pregnant makes a difference, not only to your health, but to the health of your baby.

Unfortunately, having PCOS can predispose you and your unborn baby to certain health risks (gestational diabetes, high blood pressure, pre-eclampsia and preterm delivery), but these are not inevitable, and there is much you can do – through diet – to prevent them.[1]

GESTATIONAL DIABETES

This is a form of diabetes which typically starts during pregnancy, but usually disappears once you give birth. Up to 52 per cent of women with PCOS end up with gestational diabetes, and unfortunately, half of all women who develop gestational diabetes go on to develop full blown Type 2 diabetes within ten to fifteen years of giving birth. Because you have PCOS you are already resistant to insulin, and if you don't control the problem it can tip you into gestational diabetes when you get pregnant.

Gestational diabetes can put you at greater risk of developing high blood pressure during the pregnancy, increase your chance of needing a Caesarean section and make it very likely that you would give birth to a much larger baby (over 9lb or 4kg), as the higher sugar (glucose) levels in your blood make the baby grow bigger.

Preventing gestational diabetes, if you can do so, will make your pregnancy easier and safeguard your future health. Continue with the dietary recommendations outlined in Chapter 4, particularly those aimed at reducing insulin resistance and I will list the most important supplements to continue taking at the end of this chapter.

If you have had your SHBG (sex-hormone-binding globulin) levels measured (see page 27), have another look at the results because research suggests that low levels of SHBG in women with PCOS can be a predictor of gestational diabetes.[2]

It is healthier to control or reduce the chance of gestational diabetes naturally through diet, but you may already be on metformin which is often given to PCOS sufferers and is the most commonly prescribed drug for Type 2 diabetes. Some experts suggest that metformin can help to prevent gestational diabetes,[3] while other research says metformin in pregnancy is not advantageous for women with PCOS.[4] The consensus paper on treatment related to PCOS suggests that metformin should be discontinued once pregnancy is confirmed,[5] and I would recommend asking your doctor if you could stop taking it.

Certainly, good levels of specific nutrients during pregnancy can help to prevent gestational diabetes. Both zinc and selenium (two antioxidant minerals) have been found to be lower in women with gestational diabetes,[6] so make sure your antenatal supplement contains these two minerals. Also, continue with your Omega 3 supplements as these can assist in keeping insulin resistance at bay.[7]

HIGH BLOOD PRESSURE (HYPERTENSION) AND PRE-ECLAMPSIA

For reasons we still don't fully understand, if you have PCOS you will have a greater risk of developing high blood pressure or pre-eclampsia,[8] so you need to take extra care of your health during pregnancy.

Pre-eclampsia is a dangerous form of high blood pressure that strikes after twenty weeks of pregnancy. Pregnancy-induced hypertension (also known as gestational hypertension) is diagnosed if your blood pressure rises above 140/90. If traces of protein are subsequently found in your urine (and look out for other symptoms such as water retention with swelling of the hands and feet), your diagnosis will change to pre-eclampsia, which is, very unfortunately, still a major cause of death in both the mother and baby.

Your pre-eclampsia prevention plan should include plenty of rest and keeping your salt intake to a minimum (salt can trigger and exacerbate high blood pressure). Ensure your diet is rich in fruit and vegetables. Meat is thought to be one of the main culprits, mainly because it creates an inflammatory effect in the body, so substitute it as much as possible with fish and an increase in fruit and vegetables. You will be doing the best you can if you stick to my recommendation of limiting refined carbohydrates like sugar and products made with white flour such as biscuits, bread and cakes, and reducing your intake of saturated fats too. In fact, a healthy diet has been shown to be as good as, if not better than, blood-pressure-lowering drugs if your blood pressure is rising.

Women with pre-eclampsia have been shown to have high levels of an amino acid called homocysteine[9] – a toxic by-product from the breakdown of one of the essential amino acids in our body, called methionine. It should, under normal circumstances, be detoxified by the body with the help of folic acid and vitamins B6 and B12, but if your diet is deficient in these nutrients, you can end up with high levels.

Too much homocysteine has also been linked to an increased risk of heart disease because it can cause thickening and hardening of the artery walls, making the blood more likely to clot, damaging the blood vessels and contributing to a build-up of plaque. You can get a simple home finger-prick test to check your level of homocysteine from www.naturalhealthpractice.com.

Homocysteine levels have been found to be higher in people who take metformin because it causes a vitamin B12 deficiency,[10] so if you have been taking this drug, you should get your vitamin B12 levels checked.

The message is clear: don't stop taking your multivitamin and mineral supplement and ensure it contains folic acid, and the B vitamins B6 and B12. And keep going with your Omega 3 supplement. As you get to the last trimester of pregnancy, this helps with your baby's brain and eye development and also with reducing inflammation and improving blood flow to the placenta.[11] Research has shown that women with the lowest levels of Omega 3 fats were 7.6 times more likely to end up with pre-eclampsia.[12]

Calcium can be useful in reducing blood pressure in pregnancy,[13] so ensure that it's contained in your multivitamin and mineral.

PRETERM DELIVERY

PCOS puts you at greater risk of having a premature baby, but by taking really good care of yourself you can work on preventing this from happening.

Preterm birth results in 75 per cent of neonatal deaths and the majority of neonatal intensive-care admissions. And one in three survivors beyond thirty-two weeks following preterm birth then goes on to develop educational and behavioural problems by the age of seven, so anything that can be done to reduce this risk should be done.

Make sure you are taking adequate quantities of vitamin C. It has been suggested that a deficiency of vitamin C during pregnancy is a risk factor for a preterm birth as it can cause the membranes surrounding the baby to rupture prematurely (collagen is active in the maintenance of these membranes and vitamin C helps in its manufacture). Vitamin C supplementation during pregnancy has been shown to reduce the incidence of this rupture.[14]

Low fish consumption is also a strong risk factor for preterm delivery, so make sure you include plenty of fish in your diet or a fish-oil capsule.[15] The UK Food Standards Agency recommends no more than two portions of oily fish a week during pregnancy, and to limit tuna to either two fresh tuna steaks a week or four medium tins of tuna (tinned tuna does not count as an oily fish because the oils are lost in the packing process). Fish-oil supplements are fine, but not cod-liver oil because of the high level of vitamin A could be dangerous in pregnancy. (See page 165 for more about oily-fish supplements.)

Deficiencies in vitamin D in pregnancy have been linked to reduced bone growth in the baby and the possibility of a preterm birth.[16] Vitamin D is crucial for the absorption of calcium and the formation and growth of bones. It is manufactured in your skin through sunlight, but thanks to sun creams, we are increasingly deficient, so consider having your vitamin D level checked (you can get a simple home finger-prick test to check if you are vitamin D deficient from www.naturalhealthpractice.com) and make sure there is some vitamin D3 in your antenatal supplement.

Also pay attention to your zinc intake, in food or supplement form. Zinc plays a crucial role in normal growth and development. Zinc deficiency has been found in 77 per cent of mothers and has been linked to a risk of pregnancy complications and negative effects on the baby's health.[17]

Because preterm labour has been linked to vaginal infections, probiotics may provide a level of protection too.[18] I use a product called NHP Advanced Probiotic Support which contains 22 billion organisms of different species (available from your local health food shop or from www.naturalhealthpractice.com).

SUPPLEMENTS IN PREGNANCY

I recommend that women with PCOS continue taking their fertility supplement (NHP's Fertility Support for Women – see page 162) until the twelfth week of pregnancy and then change to a good antenatal supplement. This should still contain good amounts of folic acid, plus the other B vitamins, vitamins E and D, calcium, magnesium, zinc, selenium, chromium, manganese and iron. (The one I use in the clinic is NHP's Ante Natal Support available from health food shops and www.naturalhealthpractice.com.) Vitamin C and Omega 3 fish oils always need to be added in separately to ensure good, high levels.

AN IDEAL PREGNANCY SUPPLEMENT PROGRAMME
- Antenatal multivitamin and mineral – follow the dosage on the product.
- Vitamin C – take 500mg twice daily.
- Omega 3 fish oils – take a fish oil with an EPA of 770mg and DHA over 510mg daily. Always avoid cod-liver oil in pregnancy because of the high vitamin A content. If you are vegetarian and do not want to take fish oil then add in linseed (flaxseed) oil – take 1,000mg daily.
- Probiotic – take a probiotic with a level of 22 billion organisms or more twice daily.

FUTURE HEALTH OF YOUR BABY

There has been an enormous amount of research into how the womb environment (specifically your diet) can determine your baby's future health.[19] We know that it can affect the risk of heart disease because the nutrition of the mother programmes the baby's health,[20] and more importantly for PCOS is the risk of diabetes.[21]

But if you look after yourself and eat well during your pregnancy, you will not only reduce your own risk of health problems after the birth, but also benefit your baby.

A good eating and supplement plan (particularly containing Omega 3 fats) can also reduce the risk of postnatal depression.[22, 23] Omega 3 fats play a big part in the development of the central nervous system as DHA (which is contained in the Omega 3 fats) accumulates in the brain and retina and is important for cognitive, visual and behavioural function.[24]

Studies show that children of mothers who consume Omega 3 fats during pregnancy (and go on to breastfeed) perform better in terms of IQ at the age of four.[25] These Omega 3 fats are also thought to be able to reduce risk of allergic diseases such as eczema and asthma in children if the mother took them in pregnancy because they play such a large part in controlling inflammation.[26]

It is clear that eating well throughout your pregnancy will not only help to safeguard your health and weight during pregnancy and in the future, but also protect your baby's health, so I cannot overemphasize the value of paying attention to your diet and ensuring that you are getting the best nutrients possible.

CHAPTER 13

NUTRITIONAL TESTS THAT ARE USEFUL IN TREATING PCOS

The supplements and herbs I recommend in this book provide a great overall programme that many studies – and my clinical experience – have shown will help the majority of women to deal with their PCOS.

However, I've noticed over the years that some women turn out to be particularly deficient in specific nutrients for one reason or another and need a more closely tailored programme. If, having read this book, you have suspicions that yours isn't perhaps a straightforward case of PCOS, if your symptoms have really got out of hand or if you are worried that you are running out of time to have a baby, it would be worth considering a few extra nutritional tests.

Most women who come to my clinic will be offered certain tests, depending on the severity of their PCOS, what their diet has been like generally and also whether they are struggling to get pregnant. But you can easily obtain a number of these tests online; a kit is sent to you, the sample is collected at home and the results come back with an explanation of what you should do to correct the deficiency or imbalance, if there is one. In conjunction with the advice in this book, this will help you to adapt your nutritional plan to meet your own individual needs. For instance, you may find that your vitamin D levels are extremely low, requiring you to take an extra supplement over and above what's already in your multivitamin and mineral. Or perhaps the balance between Omega 3 and Omega 6 fats in your system is out of kilter; if so, you will need to take much higher amounts of Omega 3 to redress this.

If you are concerned that you are not able to get the medical tests (blood and ultrasound scans – see Chapter 2) from your doctor or gynaecologist, it might be worth considering making an appointment at one of my clinics (see page 217) where they can be organized for you. As part of that consultation, you will also be offered a personalized nutritional programme at the same time.

I must emphasize that for the vast majority of women with PCOS, the diet, lifestyle and nutritional recommendations I make in this book will be enough. The changes you make will have such a powerful effect on your body that you really will notice improvements and you may even beat PCOS for ever.

But if you find you need a little bit more support, it might be worth considering some of the following tests (available by post – see Useful Resources, page 217).

VITAMIN D TEST

The benefits of vitamin D are numerous, not only in the battle to master your PCOS, but also for your general health. Good levels of vitamin D are important for protecting against:

- diabetes
- heart disease

- cancer
- joint pains
- autoimmune diseases
- fertility
- anti-ageing
- allergies.

Many people, particularly women, are deficient in vitamin D – some woefully so. I've seen lab reports for patients which show that their vitamin D levels are 'undetectable'. One reason for this deficiency is that our best natural source of vitamin D is sunlight, but these days we all try to stay out of the sun and use sunscreen (even in cosmetics and moisturizers).

The vitamin D detection test requires a tiny drop of blood from a finger prick. The procedure can be done easily at home and you then send the sample back to the lab for analysis to establish whether or not you are deficient. We should all have around 80µmol/L (in the US measured as 32ng/mL) of vitamin D. If you do turn out to be deficient, I'd recommend you take an extra vitamin D supplement for three months on top of your multivitamin and mineral, then retest to check your levels are back to normal.

There is a fashion in some areas to take really high doses of vitamin D as a way of protecting yourself against diseases such as cancer, but I have never found this necessary. An extra 400ius vitamin D taken as a liquid under the tongue (sublingually) is ideal as the absorption of the vitamin D is much faster and enables you to correct the deficiency in a shorter space of time. Taken on top of your multivitamin and mineral for three months, this should be enough to get your levels where they should be. Once the vitamin D deficiency has been corrected then just keep taking your multivitamin and mineral which contains a good amount of vitamin D.

As a fat-soluble vitamin, vitamin D is stored in your body for about sixty days (unlike vitamin C which is water-soluble and is excreted from the body after a few hours), so it would be unwise to take too much as possible side effects could include too high levels of calcium in the blood, dry mouth, headache, loss of appetite and fatigue.

OMEGA 3/6 RATIO TEST

Omega 3 fats play many key roles in your general health, but they are particularly useful in the control of PCOS symptoms. If you are trying to get pregnant, Omega 3s can be active in the fight against infertility in general, but particularly by increasing blood flow to the womb to help maintain a pregnancy and reducing your risk of premature birth. They also reduce insulin resistance, lower your risk of heart disease, improve brain function and help to ease painful periods.[1]

However, as I have explained earlier in the book, most women have far much too much Omega 6 in their diet, and not enough Omega 3. You need a healthy ratio of Omega 6 to Omega 3 but you can easily swing the ratio the wrong way if you eat lots of fried foods (vegetable oils increase Omega 6 levels), take evening primrose supplements (again, very high in Omega 6s and often taken in very high doses) or are vegetarian.

This is an important test for all women with PCOS because getting the right ratio of Omega 3 to 6 means that you are controlling inflammation, which plays such a central part in PCOS and its symptoms.

You can send off for an Omega 3/6 ratio test kit, do the simple finger-prick test at home, then send the kit back to the lab for analysis (see www.naturalhealthpractice.com). If the result shows your 3/6 balance is wrong, you will be given advice for reducing levels of Omega

6 in your diet, and you may be recommended to take a higher dose of Omega 3. So instead of taking two capsules of Omega 3 fish oil a day (containing 770mg EPA and 510mg DHA per day), you might need to take twice as much for three months. You would then repeat the test, and once the ratio is back to normal you would maintain that balance with just two capsules a day.

ADRENAL STRESS TEST

Your stress levels and your individual ability to cope with the rigours of stress (both physically and mentally) will play a large part in the control of your PCOS symptoms.

Although one really important stress hormone is adrenaline, it is so short lived in your body that it is almost impossible to test for it. However cortisol can be easily measured, and if you have been under a lot of stress and suspect this might be a particular problem for you, it might be useful to test your levels.

The adrenal stress test picks up cortisol levels in four simple saliva samples which you spread throughout the day. This will measure how your levels fluctuate throughout the day (they are normally highest in the morning, as you start the day and lowest at night when you are ready to wind down and go to bed). The test also measures levels of DHEA (dehydroepiandrosterone) which is the hormone that works to balance many of the negative effects of cortisol and improves your ability to cope with stress. It is good to have a normal reading of DHEA because research has shown that it helps to improve memory function, boost energy levels, and has an anti-weight effect by decreasing fat tissue, excess insulin and food intake.

You can get a blood test for cortisol, but it is designed to pick up only severe adrenal diseases such as Cushing's syndrome (in which cortisol is too high) and Addison's disease (too low), and is not helpful when looking at the effects of stress – as we are with PCOS.

The saliva adrenal stress test will show you how stressed you are and, depending on your results, you would be recommended to include certain nutrients such as magnesium, vitamin B5 and Siberian ginseng in higher amounts than those you might already be taking. Keeping your cortisol levels within the normal range is important, otherwise it can increase inflammation which is not good for PCOS and also gives the message to your body to put on more weight (fat), especially around your middle.

For more information on this test, which can be organized by post, go to www.naturalhealthpractice.com or see Useful Resources, page 217.

HOMOCYSTEINE TEST

Homocysteine is a toxic by-product from the breakdown of the essential amino acid methionine. It should – under normal circumstances – be detoxified by the body with the help of folic acid, vitamin B6 and vitamin B12. However, if you have PCOS, you are unlikely to be getting enough of these B vitamins and you may, as a consequence, end up with high levels of homocysteine. This makes it a useful marker to look out for.

Testing homocysteine levels is especially important if you are or have been on the drug metformin as it can cause a vitamin B12 deficiency.[2] As this is one of the vitamins needed to detoxify homocysteine, a deficiency would show up on a test as a high homocysteine reading.

If you are also keen to get pregnant, it is probably worth having your homocysteine levels checked, as high levels could increase your risk of the high blood pressure condition, pre-eclampsia[3] (see page

185). This is due to the fact that homocysteine can damage blood vessels and make blood more likely to clot.

There is also a link between high homocysteine levels and insulin resistance. If you find your reading is high, homocysteine can be lowered by taking extra folic acid and the vitamins B6 and B12, and this should improve insulin resistance.[4]

The homocysteine test is another simple finger-prick test that can be done at home (request a kit from www.naturalhealthpractice.com or see Useful Resources, page 217) and the sample is then sent back to the lab.

CHAPTER 14

SAFEGUARDING YOUR FUTURE HEALTH

Even if by following all the recommendations in this book you see a huge drop in your PCOS symptoms, you should still continue to closely monitor and manage your health and lifestyle.

Your symptoms may have gone and, thanks to all the changes you've made to your diet and lifestyle, you should see a return (or establishment) of a regular cycle once more, but don't forget that you still have PCOS. It can often be reversed, but you are always, unfortunately, going to be susceptible to it returning if your diet becomes unhealthy – and this means you are more at risk of certain other conditions than women without PCOS. Be alert to the risks and regard my nutritional plan as a long-term strategy, not a short-term quick fix.

There is no getting away from the fact that women who have PCOS are at greater risk of conditions like diabetes, heart disease, stroke, Alzheimer's and some cancers. It sounds like grim news, but if you manage to keep your blood-sugar levels under control (by following my recommendations) you should be able to reduce your output of insulin. This means you will be doing the best you can to reduce the harmful inflammatory response the body sets up to deal with all the excess insulin that it regards as an invader. It is this 'inflammation' that has possibly the most dangerous implications for your long-term health.

Scientists now think that inflammation is the main driving force behind many of our health problems – whether you have PCOS or not – so by controlling that you really can reduce the risk of major illnesses in later life. As you already know, if you have PCOS you will be producing more inflammation than most people,[1] so that is why controlling inflammation is so important.

Although PCOS does increase your risk of various long-term diseases and conditions, I must emphasize, it is certainly not inevitable that you will end up with these or any other health problems. If you do whatever you can to make your body more sensitive to insulin and put in place my dietary, supplement and exercise suggestions, you really can prevent many of these problems from ever developing.

HEALTH RISK: DIABETES
SOLUTION: CONTROL BLOOD-SUGAR LEVELS

The insulin resistance that blights the vast majority of women with PCOS does, unfortunately put you at increased risk of getting diabetes in later life. In fact, some experts believe the link is so strong that we should think of PCOS as a pre-diabetic state because up to 20 per cent of women with PCOS run the risk of becoming diabetic.

Your risk increases further if you:

- have a family history of Type 2 diabetes
- are aged over forty
- have gestational diabetes while pregnant
- are overweight (with a BMI of over 30).

However, the good news is that the Diabetes Prevention Program has shown that exercise and diet are nearly twice as effective as metformin at reducing the chance of developing diabetes[2] in people who are at high risk. So if you're worried about diabetes, and particularly if you have any of the extra risk factors above, it is very important to follow all the diet and exercise recommendations in this book. Do make a point of following the simple tips on pages 91–3, such as including almonds in your diet. Research on people with pre-diabetes has shown that just 2oz (50g) of almonds a day improves insulin sensitivity and lowers LDL ('bad' cholesterol).[3]

HEALTH RISK: HEART DISEASE
SOLUTION: CONTROL INSULIN RESISTANCE

If you have uncontrolled PCOS, you are also statistically at risk of developing high blood pressure, stroke and heart disease. Linked together, this combination of risks is known as metabolic syndrome, because a number of metabolic factors are thrown out of kilter by your insulin resistance. It can lead to a highly unhealthy combination of fat around your middle, high blood-sugar levels, high blood pressure, high triglyceride levels (blood fats) and low levels of HDL.

Being insulin resistant can increase your risk of a number of illnesses, as shown by the wheel on page 202. But if you work hard to keep your blood sugar under control you will be doing the best you can to help prevent diabetes and also to balance your cholesterol levels because we know that sugar intake is linked to negative changes in cholesterol, reducing levels of HDL (good) and raising levels of LDL (bad).[4]

Make sure too, that no matter how well you feel, and how under control your PCOS symptoms become, you never stop taking your good-quality multivitamin and multimineral. Keep levels of the B vitamins high to support your body in winning the battle against

INSULIN RESISTANCE AND RELATED HEALTH ISSUES

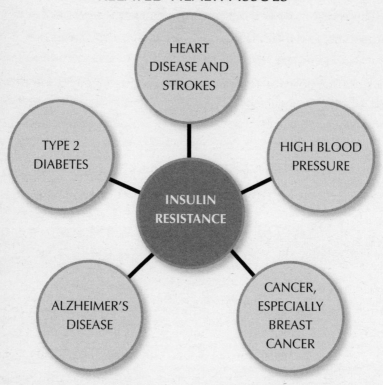

homocysteine (see pages 185–6), high levels of which have been linked to heart disease, stroke, Alzheimer's and osteoporosis, all of which become more common as we get older.

There is also some indication that the higher your insulin levels, the higher will be your homocysteine levels. In one study people with the metabolic syndrome were given both folic acid and vitamin B12. This combination not only reduced homocysteine levels, as one would expect, but also improved insulin resistance.[5] It seems that the lower the level of homocysteine, the lower the level of insulin.

You should be particularly vigilant with your B vitamins if you are taking (or have taken) the drug metformin, which causes vitamin B12 deficiency which, in turn, can create a high homocysteine level.[6]

If you are concerned, ask your GP to check your levels of vitamin B12 (or we can do this in the clinic). Also, consider a homocysteine test. This is easy to do and is just a finger-prick test performed at home and then sent to the lab. Go to www.naturalhealthpractice.com or see Useful Resources, page 217.

Do not let up with the regular exercise, as inactivity can lower homocysteine levels as you get older.[7]

HEALTH RISK: CANCERS
SOLUTION: MAINTAIN A HEALTHY WEIGHT

For everyone – whether they have PCOS or not – the risk of cancer increases with age. Unfortunately, if you have insulin resistance, your risk may be higher still.

This is because insulin is a 'grower'; it is classed as an anabolic steroid, which means that it can encourage cells to mutate and it can block a process called apoptosis, which stops cells dying. This means that some cells don't die when they should, but continue dividing and mutating. High levels of insulin have been linked to a number of different cancers including bowel, liver, pancreas, breast, ovary and womb.[8]

Women with PCOS can also have a four-fold increased risk of womb (endometrial) cancer.[9] And one study found that women with high insulin levels had a three-fold increased risk of breast cancer.[10]

The weight gain so typical of PCOS also contributes to the risk because weight is now acknowledged as an added factor with breast cancer.[11] The worst place to have extra weight is around your middle – again another trait painfully exacerbated by PCOS. One study showed that women who put on fat around their middle after the menopause are 88 per cent more likely to get breast cancer[12] because fat cells in that area become a manufacturing plant for oestrogen.

If you are concerned, check your waist-to-hip measurement (see page 88). But, once more, if you are following my recommendations, you should lose weight – particularly around your middle. And that won't just make you look better – you can be confident that it will significantly boost your long-term health and reduce your risk of serious illness and disease too.

We should include one piece of good news for women with PCOS...

THE MENOPAUSE

My aim throughout this book has been to help you reduce or even reverse the symptoms of PCOS, but you may find it interesting to know that as you get closer to the menopause, your periods could naturally become more regular and the debilitating symptoms that have blighted you for years may start to tail off.

You should go through the menopause at around the same age as a woman without PCOS (in the UK the average age is fifty-one). But be warned, research does show that postmenopausal women with PCOS can be at greater risk of heart disease and stroke.[13]

If you are very unlucky, and find your PCOS persists after menopause, you could find you still have problems with blood-sugar imbalances, excess male hormones and chronic inflammation.[14] But the measures in this book will certainly help then, just as they do now.

On a positive note, your bone-mineral density may be higher than other women and you may have a lower risk of osteoporosis and fractures, as you get older. This is because you will have had higher levels of oestrogen and androgens over the years and both these hormones will have helped to maintain good bone density.[15] Ensure that you still look after your bone health by eating well and exercising and making sure you are getting enough bone nutrients such as calcium, magnesium and vitamin D.

The other positive news is that all your concerns about an unhealthy waist-hip ratio should diminish after menopause. Although women with PCOS tend to have a higher waist-to-hip ratio generally, after the menopause women without PCOS also tend to have weight gain around the middle, so the difference – and therefore the relative health risks – between the two groups of women disappears.[16]

I have written in detail about how to look after yourself through the menopause in my book *Natural Solutions to Menopause*, which gives you information about HRT, prevention of osteoporosis and how to deal with the symptoms of the menopause (such as hot flushes and night sweats) using natural approaches.

If you have, or had PCOS, your journey through the menopause will be the same as for any woman, so it may be useful for you to know the choices you have at this natural stage in your life – how much you can minimize symptoms and ease the way through diet, exercise and supplements.

CHAPTER 15

BEYOND PCOS

By the time you get to this part of the book, I very much hope that you will have been inspired to take on board many of my recommendations. My methods absolutely work. And if you try them, it won't be long before you start to see very positive results.

I know it's not easy to make dramatic changes to your diet, particularly if you've tried diets before, and they haven't seemed to work. But every change that you make will pay off not just in terms of controlling your PCOS symptoms but for your overall health now and in the future.

Through taking on board my suggestions, you will be doing the best you possibly can to understand PCOS and how it affects you. PCOS can be managed, treated and even reversed – all naturally, without drugs, side effects and invasive procedures, and in a way that will not do anything to adversely affect the delicate balance of your body. And if you've been told you may never get pregnant – don't listen! The countless women who use my methods will tell you that if you can settle erratic hormones naturally, your fertility will start to fall into place and successful conception and healthy pregnancy can be a reality, not a dream.

You really have got nothing to lose. The sooner you control your PCOS symptoms using natural solutions, the better chance you have of protecting yourself against the potentially long-term damage that PCOS can have on your health.

You can get your life back, your femininity and your self-esteem. You just have to make that leap of faith. Your life and your health are in your hands.

I wish you well on your road to a healthy and happy life that is free of PCOS symptoms and full of good fertility.

Good luck.

Marilyn

APPENDIX I

CRITERIA FOR DIAGNOSING PCOS

There is still some confusion within the medical profession as to the criteria for diagnosing PCOS and this means that you may be told you have PCOS by one doctor and not by another.

I would suggest that you should always be tested for PCOS if you have irregular periods (longer than thirty-six days) or none at all, infertility, excess hair or acne.

At the time of going to press, there are three sets of criteria (see below) in the medical literature for the diagnosis of PCOS and I have set them out here so you can be fully informed:

1. *National Institute of Child Health and Human Development (NICHD) Criteria (1990)*

For a diagnosis of PCOS you have to have both:

- infrequent ovulation
- signs (either through physical appearance, like hirsutism or acne, or from blood tests) of high levels of male hormones.

2. Rotterdam Criteria – suggested by the European Society of Human Reproduction and Embryology (ESHRE) and the American Society for Reproductive Medicine (ASRM) (2003)

For a diagnosis of PCOS you have to have two out of:

- infrequent or no ovulation
- signs (either physical appearance – hirsutism or acne – or blood tests) of high levels of male hormones
- polycystic ovaries as seen on an ultrasound scan.

Any other possible diagnosis for the symptoms – e.g. premature menopause, Cushing's syndrome, androgen-secreting tumours – also has to be excluded.

3. Androgen Excess and PCOS Society Guidelines (2006)

For a diagnosis of PCOS you have to have both:

- signs of excess male hormones, either in the form of hirsutism or high male hormones on a blood test
- infrequent or no ovulation and/or polycystic ovaries on ultrasound scanning.

Any other possible diagnosis for the symptoms – e.g. Cushing's syndrome, androgen-secreting tumours – also has to be excluded.

The Rotterdam criteria seem to be the most widely accepted at present because they allow for women who have a milder form of PCOS and are not generally overweight to be categorized as having PCOS. Using the Rotterdam criteria, there are now four different groups of women who can all be classed as having PCOS:

- Women who have polycystic ovaries as seen on an ultrasound scan, male hormone symptoms and infrequent periods.

- Women who have polycystic ovaries as seen on an ultrasound scan and male hormone symptoms, but normal menstrual cycles.
- Women who have polycystic ovaries as seen on an ultrasound scan, no male hormone symptoms, but irregular or no periods.
- Women whose ovaries appear normal on a scan and have male hormone symptoms and irregular or no periods.

This shows just how greatly PCOS symptoms can vary from one woman to another. It also shows that even if your symptoms are very mild you may still have PCOS and should be treated as such.

APPENDIX II

FOOD NUTRIENT SOURCES

Antioxidants
Apples, avocado, berries, broccoli, cauliflower, citrus fruits, kidney beans, nuts and seeds, oily fish, tomatoes, vegetable oils, whole grains

Beta-carotene
Butternut squash, carrots, dark green leafy vegetables, mango, papaya, peaches, peppers, sweet potato, tomatoes, watermelon

Biotin
Almonds, cabbage, cauliflower, cherries, eggs, grapefruit, herring, lettuce, oysters, peas, sweetcorn, tomatoes, watermelon

Calcium (non-dairy)
Almonds, amaranth, black beans, broccoli, brown rice, buckwheat, cabbage, chickpeas, eggs, figs, hazelnuts, parsley, pinto beans, quinoa, sardines (tinned with edible bones), spring greens, seaweed, sesame seeds, sunflower seeds, soya, tahini, walnuts, watercress, wild salmon (tinned with edible bones)

Chromium
Apples, eggs, green peppers, oysters, parsnips, potatoes, rye

Folic acid
Asparagus, broccoli, Brussels sprouts, cashew nuts, cauliflower, sesame seeds, spinach, walnuts

Iodine
Fish, seaweed (dulse, nori, wakame)

Iron (non-meat)
Beetroot, dried apricots, molasses, parsley, prunes, pumpkin seeds, spinach, watercress

Magnesium
Apricots, broccoli, dark green leafy vegetables, figs, kale, nuts, prunes, pumpkin, sesame seeds, spinach, watercress

Manganese
Beetroot, blackberries, celery, endive, grapes, lettuce, oats, raspberries, watercress

Omega 3 (essential fatty acid)
Dark green leafy vegetables, flaxseeds (linseeds) and flaxseed oil, herring, mackerel, mustard seeds, pilchards, rapeseed oil, sardines, soya, tuna, walnuts, wild salmon

Omega 6 (essential fatty acid)
Almonds, flaxseeds (linseeds) and flaxseed oil, hemp seeds and hemp oil, pumpkin seeds, sunflower seeds, walnuts, wheatgerm

Phytoestrogens
Alfalfa sprouts, chickpeas, fennel, flaxseed (linseed), lentils, miso, mung beans, parsley, sage, sesame seeds, soya milk, tamari (gluten-free soy sauce), tempeh, tofu

Protein sources (non-meat)
Cheese, fish, eggs, natural yogurt, nuts and seeds, pulses, quinoa, soya milk, tofu

Selenium
Brazil nuts, brown rice, cod, molasses, oats, seafood, tuna

Superfoods
Allium family (garlic, onions, leeks and chives), apricot kernels, blue-berries, broccoli, butternut squash, goji berries, pomegranate, quinoa, seaweed (dulse, nori, wakame), sprouted beans, sweet potato

Vitamin A (retinol)
Dairy produce, eggs

Vitamin B1 (Thiamin)
Asparagus, beans, Brussels sprouts, cabbage, cauliflower, courgette, lettuce, mushrooms, peas, peppers, squash, tomatoes, watercress

Vitamin B2 (Riboflavin)
Asparagus, bamboo shoots, bean sprouts, broccoli, cabbage, mackerel, mushrooms, pumpkin, tomatoes, watercress

Vitamin B3 (Niacin)
Asparagus, cabbage, courgettes, mackerel, mushrooms, salmon, squash, tomatoes, tuna

Vitamin B5 (Pantothenic acid)
Alfalfa sprouts, avocado, broccoli, cabbage, celery, eggs, lentils, mushrooms, peas, squash, strawberries, tomatoes, watercress

Vitamin B6 (Pyridoxine)
Asparagus, bananas, broccoli, Brussels sprouts, cabbage, cauliflower, kidney beans, lentils, onions, peppers, seeds and nuts, squash, watercress

Vitamin B12 (Cyanocobalamin)
Cheese, eggs, oysters, sardines, shrimp, tuna

Vitamin C
Blackcurrants, broccoli, cabbage, cauliflower, grapefruit, kiwi fruit, lemons, limes, melon, oranges, peppers, strawberries, watercress

Vitamin D
Cottage cheese, eggs, herring, mackerel, oysters, salmon

Vitamin E
Almonds, asparagus, avocado, cabbage, cashews, hazelnuts, lentils, mung beans, olive oil, olives, peas, sardines, sesame seeds, spinach, sunflower seeds, wild salmon

Zinc
Alfalfa, almonds, Brazil nuts, mung beans, oats, oysters, pecans, prawns, pumpkin seeds, sesame seeds, sunflower seeds, walnuts, wheatgerm

USEFUL RESOURCES

THE DR MARILYN GLENVILLE PHD CLINICS
Consultation
All of the qualified nutritionists who work in my three UK clinics (and two in Ireland) have been trained by me in my specific approach to women's healthcare including, of course, PCOS and fertility.

Clinics are located at:

UK
- Viveka, St John's Wood, London
- The Medical Chambers, Kensington, London
- The Dr Marilyn Glenville Clinic, Tunbridge Wells, Kent

To book a personal or telephone appointment at any of these clinics, or for more information, please contact us at:

The Dr Marilyn Glenville Clinic
14 St John's Road
Tunbridge Wells
Kent TN4 9NP
Tel: 0870 5329244/Fax: 0870 5329255
Int. Tel: +44 1 892 515905/Fax: +44 1 892 515914
Email: health@marilynglenville.com
Website: www.marilynglenville.com

Ireland

• Positive Nutrition, Dublin and Galway

To book a personal or telephone appointment at either of these clinics, or for more information, please contact us on:

Tel: 01 402 0777
Website: www.positivenutrition.ie

Supplements and tests

For more information about or to order any of the supplements and tests mentioned in this book go to:

The Natural Health Practice (NHP)
Tel: 0845 8800915
Int. Tel: + 44 1 892 507598
Website: www.naturalhealthpractice.com

The Natural Health Practice stocks only the highest-quality, most effective nutritional supplements and natural products that have my personal approval and is my 'Supplier of Choice'.

Workshops and talks

For a list of my forthcoming workshops and talks, please see my website www.marilynglenville.com. If you would like me to come and give a workshop or talk near you, please call my clinic for information about how to arrange it.

Free health tips

If you would like to receive my exclusive Health Tips by email, drop me a line at health@marilynglenville.com. Just mention 'Free Health Tips' in the subject line and you will be added to my special list to receive regular health tips and other useful information.

NOTES

Chapter 1: What is PCOS?

1. Eisner, J.R. *et al.*, 'Ovarian hyperandrogenism in adult female rhesus monkeys exposed to prenatal androgen excess', *Fertil Steril*, 77 (2002), 167–72

2. Vrbikova, J. *et al.*, 'Insulin sensitivity in women with polycystic ovary syndrome', *J Clin Endocrinol Metab*, 89 (2004), 6, 2942–5

3. Carmina, E. *et al.*, 'Does ethnicity influence the prevalence of adrenal hyper-androgenism and insulin resistance in PCOS', *Am J Obstet Gynaecol*, 167 (1992), 1807–12

4. Kauffman, R.P. *et al.*, 'PCOS and insulin resistance in white and Mexican American women: A comparison of two distinct populations', *Am J Obstet Gynaecol*, 187 (2002), 1362–9

5. Wijeyaratne, C.N. *et al.*, 'Clinical manifestations and insulin resistance in PCOS among South Asians and Caucasians: is there a difference?' *Clin Endocrinol*, 57 (2002), 343–50

6. Farrow, A. *et al.*, 'Prolonged use of oral contraception before a planned pregnancy is associated with a decreased risk of delayed conception', *Hum Reprod*, 17 (2002),10, 2754–61

7. Diamanti-Kandarakis, E. *et al.*, 'A modern medical quandary: PCOS, insulin resistance and oral contraceptive pills', *J Clin Endocrinol Metab*, 88 (2003), 5, 1927–32

Chapter 2: Diagnosing PCOS

1. Muttukrishna, S. *et al.*, 'Antral follicle count, anti-mullerian hormone and inhibin B: predictors of ovarian response in assisted reproductive technology?' *BJOG*, 10 (2005), 1384–90

Chapter 3: *Your Medical Options*

1. Cagnacci, A., 'Oral contraceptives and insulin sensitivity', *Fertil Steril*, **86** (2006), 1, 5

2. Kashyap, S. *et al.*, 'Insulin-sensitising agents as primary therapy for patients with polycystic ovarian syndrome', *Hum Reprod*, **19** (2004), 2474–83

3. Knowler, W.C. *et al.*, 'Ten year follow up of diabetes incidence and weight loss in the Diabetes Prevention Program Outcome Study', *Lancet*, **374** (2009), 1677–86

4. Fux Otta, C., 'Clinical, metabolic, and endocrine parameters in response to metformin and lifestyle intervention in women with polycystic ovary syndrome: A randomized, double-blind, and placebo control trial', *Gynaecol Endocrinol*, **8** (2009), 1–6

5. Costello, M. *et al.*, 'Insulin-sensitising drugs versus the combined oral contraceptive Pill for hirsutism, acne and risk of diabetes, cardiovascular disease, and endometrial cancer in polycystic ovary syndrome', *Cochrane Database Syst Rev*, **24** (2007), 1, CD005552

6. Luque-Ramirez, M. and Escobar-Morreale, H.F., 'Treatment of PCOS with metformin ameliorates insulin resistance in parallel with the decrease of serum interleukin-6 concentrations', *Horm Metab Res*, **42** (2010), 11, 815–20

7. Ascer, E. *et al.*, 'Atorvastatin reduces proinflammatory markers in hypercholesterolemic patients', *Atherosclerosis*, **177** (2004), 1, 161–6

8. Kazerooni, T. *et al.*, 'Effects of metformin plus simvastatin on PCOS: a prospective, randomised double blind, placebo controlled study', *Fertil Steril*, **94** (2010), 6, 2208–13

9. de Jager, J. *et al.*, 'Long term treatment with metformin in patients with type 2 diabetes and risk of vitamin B12 deficiency: randomised placebo controlled trial', *BMJ*, **340** (2010), *c*. 2181

10. Ting, R.Z. *et al.*, 'Risk factors of vitamin B12 deficiency in patients receiving metformin', *Arch Intern Med*, **166** (2006), 18, 1975–9

Chapter 4: *The Seven-step Diet to Beat PCOS*

1. Gialluria, F. et al., 'Androgens in PCOS: the role of exercise and diet', *Semin Reprod Med*, **27** (2009), 4, 306–15; and Marsh, K.A., 'Effect of a low glycemic index compared with a conventional healthy diet on PCOS', *Am J Clin Nutr*, **92** (2010), 83–92; and Chavarro, J.E. *et al.*, 'Diet and lifestyle in the prevention of ovulatory disorder infertility', *Obstet Gynecol*, **110** (2007), 5, 1050–8; and O'Connor, A. *et al.*, 'Metabolic and hormonal aspects of PCOS: the impact of diet', *Proc Nut Soc*, **69** (2010), 4, 628–35

2. Vrbikova, J. *et al.*, 'Insulin sensitivity in women with polycystic ovary syndrome', *J Clin Endocrinol Metab*, **89** (2004), 6, 2942–5

3. Marsh, K.A. *et al.*, 'Effect of a low glycemic index compared with a conventional healthy diet on PCOS', *Am J Clin Nutr*, **92** (2010), 83–92

4. Bazzano, L.A. *et al.*, 'Intake of fruit, vegetables and fruit juices and risk of diabetes in women', *Diabetes Care*, **31** (2008), 7, 1311–17

5. Chandalia, M. *et al.*, 'Beneficial effects of high dietary fiber intake in patients with type 2 diabetes mellitus', *NEJM*, **342** (2000), 1392–8

6. Jayagopal, V. *et al.*, 'Beneficial effects of soy phytoestrogen intake in postmenopausal women with type 2 diabetes', *Diabetes Care*, **25** (2002), 1709–14

7. Welsh, J.A. *et al.*, 'Caloric sweetener consumption and dyslipidemia among US adults', *JAMA*, **303** (2010), 15, 1490–97

8. Blundell, J.E. and Hill, A.J.,'Paradoxical effects of an intense sweetener (aspartame) on appetite', *Lancet*, **1** (1986), 8489, 1092–3

9. Keast, D.R. *et al.*, 'Snacking is associated with reduced risk of overweight and reduced abdominal obesity in adolescents: National Health and Nutrition Examination Survey (NHANES) 1999–2004', *Am J Clin Nutr*, **92** (2010), 4280435

10. Yashodhara, B.M. *et al.*, 'Omega 3 fatty acids: a comprehensive review of their role in health and disease', *Postgrad Med J*, **85** (2009), 1000, 84–90

11. Liepa, G.U. *et al.*, 'PCOS and other androgen excess related conditions: can changes in dietary intake make a difference?' *Nutr Clin Pract*, **23** (2008), 1, 63–71

12. Phelan, N., *et al.*, 'Hormonal and metabolic effects of polyunsaturated fatty acids in young women with polycystic ovary syndrome: results from a cross-sectional analysis and a randomized, placebo-controlled, crossover trial', *Am J Clin Nutr*, **93** (2011), 3, 652–62

13. Pham, A.Q. *et al.*, 'Cinnamon supplementation in patients with type 2 diabetes mellitus', *Pharmacotherapy*, **27** (2007), 595–9; and Kirkham, S. *et al.*, 'The potential of cinnamon to reduce blood glucose levels in patients with type 2 diabetes and insulin resistance', *Diabetes Obes Metab*, **11** (2009), 12, 1100–13

14. Wang, J.G. *et al.*, 'The effect of cinnamon extract on insulin resistance parameters in PCOS: a pilot study', *Fertil Steril*, **88** (2007), 240–3

15. Qin, B. *et al.*, 'Cinnamon: potential role in the prevention of insulin resistance, metabolic syndrome and type 2 diabetes', *J Diabetes Sci Technol*, **4** (2010), 3, 685

16. Therry van Dessel, H.J. *et al.*, 'Elevated serum levels of free insulin-like growth factor 1 in PCOS', *J Clin Endocrinol Metabol*, **84** (1999), 3030–35

17. Wu, X.K. *et al.*, 'Selective ovary resistance to insulin signalling in women with PCOS', *Fertil Steril*, **80** (2003), 4, 954–65

18. Gialauria, F. *et al.*, 'Androgens in PCOS: the role of exercise and diet', *Semin Reprod Med*, **27** (2009), 4, 306–15

19. Ostman, E.M. *et al.*, 'Inconsistency between glycemic and insulinemic responses to regular and fermented milk products', *Am J Clin Nutr*, **74** (2001), 1, 96–100

20. Liljeberg, E. *et al.*, 'Milk as a supplement to mixed meals may elevate post-prandial insulinemia', *Eur J Clin Nutri*, **55** (2001), 11, 994–9

21. Larsson, S.C. *et al.*, 'Milk, milk products and lactose intake and ovarian cancer risk: A meta-analysis of epidemiological studies', *Int J Cancer*, **118** (2006), 2, 431–41

22. Smith, R. *et al.*, 'The effect of a high protein, low glycemic load diet versus a conventional, high glycemic load diet on biochemical parameters associated with acne vulgaris', *J Am Acad Dermatol*, **57** (2007), 2, 247–56

23. Butler, G. *et al.*, 'Fat composition of organic and conventional retail milk in northeast England', *J Dairy Sci*, **94** (2011), 1, 24–36

24. Barnard, N.D. *et al.*, 'Diet and SHBG, dysmenorrhoea and premenstrual symptoms', *Obstet Gynecol*, **95** (2000), 2, 245–50

25. Low, Y.L. *et al.*, 'Phytoestrogen exposure is associated with circulating sex hormones levels in postmenopausal women and interact with ESR1 and NR1I2 gene variants', *Cancer Epidemiol Biomarkers Prev*, **16** (2007), 5, 1009–16

26. Wu, A.H. *et al.*, 'Dietary patterns and breast cancer risk in Asian American women', *Am J Clin Nutr*, **89** (2009), 4, 145–54

27. Chen, M.J. *et al.*, 'Low sex hormone-binding globulin is associated with low high-density lipoprotein cholesterol and metabolic syndrome in women with PCOS', *Human Reproduction*, **21** (2006), 2266–71

28. Hamed, S. *et al.*, 'Red wine consumption improves in vitro migration of endothelial progenitor cells in young, healthy individuals', *Am J Clin Nutr*, **92** (2010), 1, 161–9

29. Roelfsema, F. *et al.*, 'Cortisol production rate is similarly elevated in obese women with or without the PCOS', *J Clin Endocrinol Metab*, **95** (2010), 7, 3318–24

30. Lin, J. *et al.*, 'Green tea polyphenols epigallocatechin gallate inhibits adipogenesis and induces apoptosis in 3T3-L1 adipocytes', *Obes Res*, **13** (2005), 6, 982–90

31. Ibid.

32. Wu, A.H., 'Tea and circulating oestrogen levels in postmenopausal Chinese women in Singapore', *Carcinogenesis*, **26** (2005), 5, 976–80

33. Hininger-Favier, I. *et al.*, 'Green tea extract decreases oxidative stress and improves insulin sensitivity in an animal model of insulin resistance, the fructose-fed rat', *J Am Coll Nutr*, **28** (2009), 4, 355–61

34. Simopoulos, A.P., 'Evolutionary aspects of diet: the omega-6/omega-3 ratio and the brain', *Mol Neurobiol*, **44** (2011), 2, 203–15

35. Escobar-Morreale, H.F., 'Circulating inflammatory markers in PCOS: a systematic review and meta-analysis', *Fertil Steril*, **95** (2011), 3, 1048–58

36. Chavarro, J.E. *et al.*, 'Dietary fatty acid intakes and the risk of ovulatory infertility', *Am J Clin Nutr*, **85** (2007), 1, 231–7

37. Kavanagh, K. *et al.*, 'Trans fat diet induces abdominal obesity and changes in insulin sensitivity in monkeys', *Obesity*, **15** (2007), 1675–84

38. Salmeron, J. *et al.*, 'Dietary fat intake and risk of type 2 diabetes in women', *Am J Clin Nutr*, **73** (2001), 6, 1019–26

39. Calder, P.C. *et al.*, 'Inflammatory disease processes and interactions with nutrition', *B J Nutr*, **101** (2009), Supp 1–45

40. Takiishi, T. *et al.*, 'Vitamin D and diabetes', *Endocrinol Metab Clin North Am*, **39** (2010), 2, 419–46

41. Pearce, S.H. and Cheetham, T.D., 'Diagnosis and management of vitamin D deficiency', *BMJ*, **340** (2010), 7738, 142–7

42. Nowson, C.A. and Margerison, C., 'Vitamin D intake and vitamin D status of Australians', *Med J Aust*, **177** (2002), 3, 149–52

Chapter 5: How to Use Supplements and Herbs

1. *The Independent Food Commission's Food Magazine*, 2005

2. Yeh, G.Y. *et al.*, 'Systematic review of herbs and dietary supplements for glycemic control in diabetes', *Diabetes Care*, **26** (2003), 4, 1277–94

3. Lucidi, R.S. *et al.*, 'Effect of chromium supplementation on insulin resistance and ovarian and menstrual cyclicity in women with PCOS', *Fertil Steril*, **84** (2005), 6, 1755–7

4. 'A scientific review: the role of chromium in insulin resistance', *Diabetes Educ*, (2004), Supp 2–14

5. Singer, G.M. and Geohas, J., 'The effect of chromium picolinate and biotin supplementation on glycemic control in poorly controlled patients with type 2 diabetes mellitus: a placebo-controlled, double-blinded, randomised trial', *Diabetes Technol Ther*, **8** (2006), 6, 636–43

6. Grundy, S.M. *et al.*, 'Efficacy, safety and tolerability of once daily niacin for the treatment of dyslipidemia associated with Type 2 diabetes', *Arch Intern Med*, **162** (2002), 1568–76

7. de Jager, J. *et al.*, 'Long term treatment with metformin in patients with type 2 diabetes and risk of vitamin B12 deficiency: randomised placebo controlled trial', *BMJ*, **340** (2010), c.2181

8. Nestler, J.E. *et al.*, 'Ovulatory and metabolic effects of D-chiro-inositol in the PCOS', *NEJM*, **340** (1999), 17, 1314–20; and Iuorno, M.J. *et al.*, 'Effects of d-chiro-inositol in lean women with the PCOS', *Endocr Pract*, **8** (2002), 6, 417–23

9. Gerli, S. *et al.*, 'Effects of inositol on ovarian function and metabolic factors in women with PCOS: a randomised double blind placebo controlled trial', *Eur Rev Med Pharmacol Sci*, **7** (2003), 6, 151–9

10. Michos, E.D., 'Vitamin D deficiency and the risk of incident Type 2 diabetes', *Future Cardiology J*, **5** (2009), 1, 15–18

11. Chowdhury, T.A. *et al.*, 'Vitamin D and Type 2 diabetes: Is there a link?' *Prim Care Diabetes*, **3** (2009), 2, 115–16

12. Knekt, P. *et al.*, 'Serum vitamin D and subsequent occurrence of Type 2 diabetes', *Epidem*, **19** (2008), 5, 666–71

13. Hahn, S. *et al.*, 'Low serum 25-hydroxyvitamin D concentrations are associated with insulin resistance and obesity in women with polycystic ovary syndrome', *Exp Clin Endocrinol Diabetes*, **114** (2006), 10, 577–83

14. Thys-Jacobs, S. *et al.*, 'Vitamin D and calcium dysregulation in the PCOS', *Steroids*, **64** (1999), 6, 430–35

15. Takaya, J. *et al.*, 'Intracellular magnesium and insulin resistance', *Magnes Res*, **17** (2004), 2, 126–36

16. Song, Y. *et al.*, 'Dietary magnesium intake in relation to plasma insulin levels and risk of Type 2 diabetes in women', *Diabetes Care*, **27** (2004), 1, 59–65

17. Chen, M.D. *et al.*, 'Zinc may be a mediator of leptin production in humans', *Life Sci*, **66** (2000), 22, 2143–9

18. Hodgson, J.M., Watts, G.F., Playford, D.A. *et al*, 'Coenzyme Q10 improves blood pressure and glycaemic control: a controlled trial in subjects with type 2 diabetes', *Eur J Clin Nutr*, **56** (2002), 11, 1137–42

19. El Midaoui, A. and de Champlain, J., 'Prevention of hypertension, insulin resistance and oxidative stress by alpha-lipoic acid', *Hypertension*, **39** (2002), 2, 303–7

20. Phelan, N. *et al.*, 'Hormonal and metabolic effects of polyunsaturated fatty acids in young women with polycystic ovary syndrome: results from a

cross-sectional analysis and a randomized, placebo-controlled, crossover trial', *Am J Clin Nutr*, **93** (2011), 3, 652–62

21. Kurduoglu, Z. *et al.*, 'Oxidative status and its relation with insulin resistance in young non-obese women with PCOS', *J Endrocrinol Invest* (2011), April 26

22. Harding, A.H. *et al.*, 'Plasma vitamin C level, fruit and vegetable consumption, and the risk of new-onset type 2 diabetes mellitus: the European prospective investigation of cancer – Norfolk prospective study', *Arch Intern Med*, **168** (2008),14, 1493–9

23. Johnston, C.S., 'Strategies for healthy weight loss: from vitamin C to the glycemic response', *J Am Coll Nutr*, **24** (2005), 3, 158–65

24. Fulghesu, A.M. *et al.*, 'N-acetyl-cysteine treatment improves insulin sensitivity in women with polycystic ovary syndrome', *Fertil Steril*, **77** (2002), 6, 1128–35

25. Nasr, A., 'Effect of N-acetyl-cysteine after ovarian drilling in clomiphene citrate-resistant PCOS women: a pilot study', *Reprod Biomed Online*, **20** (2009), 3, 403–9

26. Masha, A. *et al.*, 'Prolonged treatment with N-acetylcysteine and L-arginine restores gonadal function in patients with PCOS', *J Endocrinol Invest*, **32** (2009), 11, 870–72

27. Heaney, R.P. *et al.*, 'Vitamin D(3) is more potent than Vitamin D(2) in humans', *J Clin Endocrinol Metab*, **96** (2011), 3, E447–52

28. Li-Qiang, Q. *et al.*, 'Higher branched chain amino acid intake is associated with a lower prevalence of being overweight or obese in middle aged East Asian and Western adults', *J Nutr*, **141** (2011), 2, 249–54

29. Cani, P.D. and Delzenne, N.M., 'The role of the gut microbiota in energy metabolism and metabolic disease', *Curr Pharm Des*, **15** (2009), 13, 1546–58

30. Cani, P.D. *et al.*, 'Role of gut microflora in the development of obesity and insulin resistance following high-fat diet feeding', *Pathol Biol* (Paris), **56** (2008), 5, 305–9

31. Kadooka, Y. *et al.*, 'Regulation of abdominal adiposity by probiotics (Lactobacillus gasseri SBT2055) in adults with obese tendencies in a randomized controlled trial', *Eur J Clin Nutri*, **64** (2010), 6, 636–43

32. Hininger-Favier, I, *et al.*, 'Green tea extract decreases oxidative stress and improves insulin sensitivity in an animal model of insulin resistance, the fructose-fed rat', *J Am Coll Nutr*, **28** (2009), 4, 355–61

33. Lim, C.E. and Wong, W.S., 'Current evidence of acupuncture on PCOS', *Gynecol Endocrinol*, **26** (2010), 6, 473–8

Chapter 6: *Controlling Your Weight*

1. Norman, R.J. *et al.*, 'Improving reproductive performance in overweight/ obese women with effective weight management', *Hum Reprod Update*, **10** (2004), 267–80

2. Tolino, A. *et al.*, 'Evaluation of ovarian functionality after a dietary treatment in obese women with PCOS', *Eur J Obstet Gynecol Reprod Biol*, **119** (2005), 1, 87–93; and Crosignani *et al.*, 'Overweight and obese anovulatory patients with polycystic ovaries: parallel improvement in anthropometric indices, ovarian physiology and fertility rate induced by diet', *Hum Reprod*, **18** (2003), 9, 1928–32

3. Crosignani, *et al.*, 'Overweight and obese anovulatory patients with polycystic ovaries: parallel improvement in anthropometric indices, ovarian physiology and fertility rate induced by diet', *Hum Reprod*, **18** (2003), 9, 1928–32

4. Kiddy, D.S. *et al.*, 'Improvement in endocrine and ovarian function during dietary treatment of obese women with polycystic ovary syndrome', *Clinical Endocrinology*, **36** (1992), 105–11

5. Clark, A.M. *et al.*, 'Weight loss results in significant improvement in pregnancy and ovulation rates in anovulatory obese women', *Hum Reprod*, **10** (1995) 10, 2705–12

6. Wright, C.E. *et al.*, 'Dietary intake, physical activity and obesity in women with PCOS', *Int J Obes Relat Metab Discord*, **28** (2004), 8, 1026–32

7. Hoeger, K.M., 'Role of lifestyle modification in the management of PCOS', *Best Pract Res Clin Endocrinol Metab*, **20** (2006), 2, 293–310

8. Corbett, S.J. *et al.*, 'Type 2 diabetes, cardiovascular disease and the evolutionary paradox of the polycystic ovary syndrome: a fertility first hypothesis', *Am J Hum Bio*, **21** (2009), 5, 587–98

9. Janssen, O.E., 'High prevalence of autoimmune thyroiditis in patients with PCOS', *Eur J Endocrin*, **150** (2004), 3, 363–9

10. Moran, L.J. *et al.*, 'Ghrelin and measures of satiety are altered in PCOS but not differentially affected by diet composition', *J Clin Endocrinol Metab*, **89** (2004), 7, 3337–44

11. Ertuck, *et al.*, 'Serum leptin levels correlate with obesity parameters but not with hyperinsulinism in women with PCOS', *Fertil Steril*, **82** (2004), 5, 1364–8

12. Hahn, S. *et al.*, 'Low serum 25-hydroxyvitamin D concentrations are associated with insulin resistance and obesity in women with polycystic ovary syndrome', *Exp Clin Endocrinol Diabetes*, **114** (2006), 10, 577–83

13. Hursel, R. *et al.*, 'The effects of green tea on weight loss and weight mainte-
    nance: a meta-analysis', *Int J Obes (Lond)*, **9** (2009), 956–61

14. Khan, A. *et al.*, 'Cinnamon improves glucose and lipids of people with Type
    2 diabetes', *Diabetes Care*, **26** (2003), 12, 3215–18

15. Ludvik, B. *et al.*, 'Improved metabolic control by Ipomoea batatas (Caiapo)
    is associated with increased adiponectin and decreased fibrinogen levels in
    type 2 diabetic subjects', *Diabetes Obes Metab*, **10** (2008), 7, 586–92

16. Fujioka, K. *et al.*, 'The effects of grapefruit on weight and insulin resistance:
    relationship to the metabolic syndrome', *J Med Food*, **9** (2006), 1, 49–54

17. Lundahl, J. *et al.*, 'Relationship between time of intake of grapefruit juice
    and its effect on pharmacokinetics and pharmacodynamics of felodipine in
    healthy subjects', *Eur J Clin Pharmacol*, **49** (1995), 61–70

18. Sugiyama, M. *et al.*, 'Glycemic index of single and mixed meal foods among
    common Japanese foods with white rice as a reference food', *Eur J Clin
    Nutri*, **57** (2003), 743–52

19. Liljeberg, H. and Bjorck, I., 'Delayed gastric emptying rate may explain
    improved glycaemia in healthy subjects to a starchy meal with added vine-
    gar', *Eur J Clin Nutri*, **52** (1998), 368–71

20. Harland, J.I. and Garton, L.E., 'Whole grain intake as a marker of healthy
    body weight and adiposity', *Public Health Nutr*, **11** (2008), 6, 554–63

21. Orio, F. *et al.*, 'PCOS and obesity: non pharmacological approaches',
    Minerva Ginecol, **59** (2007), 1, 63–73

22. Herriot, A.M. *et al.*, 'A retrospective audit of patients with PCOS: the effect
    of a reduced glycemic load diet', *J Hum Nutr Diet*, **21** (2008), 4, 337–45

23. Mori, A.M. *et al.*, 'Acute and second meal effects of almond form in impaired
    glucose tolerant adults: a randomised crossover trial', *Nutr Metab* (Lond), **8**
    (2011), 1, 6

24. Li, S.C. *et al.*, 'Almond consumption improved glycemic control and lipid
    profiles in patients with type 2 diabetes mellitus', *Metabolism*, **60** (2010), 4,
    474–9

25. Kalgaonkar, S. *et al.*, 'Differential effects of walnuts versus almonds on
    improving metabolic and endocrine parameters in PCOS', *Eur J Clin Nutri*,
    65 (2011), 3, 386–93

26. World Health Organization, Joint WHO/FAO Expert Consultation, 'Diet,
    Nutrition and the Prevention of Chronic Diseases', 2003, *WHO Technical
    Report Series*, 916

27. Vonk, R.J. *et al.*, 'Digestion of so-called resistant starch sources in the human
    small intestines', *Am J Clin Nutr*, **72** (2000), 432–8

28. Johnson, K.L. *et al.*, 'Resistant starch improves insulin sensitivity in metabolic syndrome', *Diabetic Medicine*, **27** (2010), 391–7

29. Wansink, B. *et al.*, 'Super bowls: serving bowl size and food consumption', *JAMA*, **293** (2005), 14, 1727–8

30. Farschchi, H.R. *et al.*, 'Beneficial metabolic effects of regular meal frequency on dietary thermogenesis, insulin sensitivity and fasting lipid profiles in healthy obese women', *Am J Clin Nutr*, **81** (2005), 1, 16–24

31. Zepeda, L. and Deal, D., *New Scientist*, 5 September 2008, page 21

32. Oldham-Cooper, R.E. *et al.*, 'Playing a computer game during lunch affects fullness, memory for lunch and later snack intake', *Am J Clin Nutr*, **93** (2011), 2, 308–13

33. Thomas, D.E. *et al.*, 'Low glycaemic index or low glycaemic load diets for overweight and obesity', *Cochrane Database Syst Rev*, **18** (2007), 3, CD005105

34. Nedeltcheva, A. *et al.*, 'Insufficient sleep undermines dietary efforts to reduce adiposity', *Ann Intern Med*, 153 (5 October 2010), 435–41

35. Donga, E. *et al.*, 'A single night of partial sleep deprivation induces insulin resistance in multiple metabolic pathways in healthy subjects', *J Clin Endocrinol Metab*, **95** (2010), 6, 2963–8

36. Spiegel, K. *et al.*, 'Impact of sleep debt on metabolic and endocrine function', *Lancet*, **354** (1999), 1435–9

37. Buman, M.P. *et al.*, 'Exercise as a treatment to enhance sleep', *Am J Lifestyle Med*, **4** (2010), 6, 500–14

38. Jayagopal, V. *et al.*, 'Orlistat is as beneficial as metformin in the treatment of polycystic ovarian syndrome', *J Clin Endocrinol Metab*, **90** (2005), 729–33

39. Sabuncu, T. *et al.*, 'Sibutramine has a positive effect on clinical and metabolic parameters in obese patients with polycystic ovary syndrome', *Fertil Steril*, **80** (2003), 1199–204

40. Tang, T. *et al.*, 'Combined lifestyle modification and metformin in obese patients with polycystic ovary syndrome. A randomized, placebo-controlled, double-blind multicentre study', *Hum Reprod*, **21** (2006), 1, 80–89

41. Thessalonki ESHRE/ASRM-sponsored PCOS Consensus Workshop Group, 'Consensus on infertility treatment related to PCOS', *Hum Reprod*, **23** (2008), 2, 462–7

42. Escobar-Morreale, H.F. *et al.*, 'The polycystic ovary syndrome associated with morbid obesity may resolve after weight loss induced by bariatric surgery', *J Clin Endocrinol Metab*, **90** (2005), 12, 6364–9

Chapter 7: Exercise

1. Palomba, S. *et al.*, 'Structured exercise training programme versus hypocaloric hyperproteic diet in obese polycystic ovary syndrome patients with anovulatory infertility: a 24-week pilot study', *Hum Reprod*, **3** (2008), 642–50

2. Palomba, S. *et al.*, 'Six weeks of structured exercise training and hypocaloric diet increases the probability of ovulation after clomiphene citrate in overweight and obese patients with polycystic ovary syndrome: a randomised controlled trial', *Hum Reprod*, **25** (2010), 11, 2783–91

3. Solomon, T.P. *et al.*, 'A low-glycemic index diet combined with exercise reduces insulin resistance, postprandial hyperinsulinemia, and glucose-dependent insulinotropic polypeptide responses in obese, prediabetic humans', *Am J Clin Nutr*, **92** (2010), 6, 1359–68, and Moran, L.J. *et al.*, 'Treatment of obesity in PCOS: a position statement of the Androgen Excess and PCOS Society', *Fertil Steril*, **92** (2009), 6, 1966–82

4. Houts, C.R. *et al.*, 'Stress, inflammation and yoga practice', *Psychom Med*, **72** (2010), 2, 113–21

5. Church, T.S. *et al.*, 'Effects of aerobic and resistance training on hemoglobin A1c levels in patients with type 2 diabetes', *JAMA*, **304** (2010), 20, 2253–62

6. Tremblay, A. *et al.*, 'Impact of exercise intensity on body fatness and skeletal muscle metabolism', *Metab Clin Exp*, **43** (1994), 7, 814–18

7. Tabata, I. *et al.*, 'Effects of moderate-intensity endurance and high-intensity intermittent training on anaerobic capacity and VO_2max', *Med Sci Sports Exerc*, **28** (1996), 10, 1327–30

8. Van Proeven, K. *et al.*, 'Training in the fasted state improves glucose tolerance during fat-rich diet', *J Physiol*, **588** (Pt 21) (2010), 4289–302

Chapter 8: Your Hair and Skin

1. de Jager, J. *et al.*, 'Long term treatment with metformin in patients with type 2 diabetes and risk of vitamin B12 deficiency: randomised placebo controlled trial', *BMJ*, **340** (2010), c.2181

2. Rushton, D.H. *et al.*, 'Causes of hair loss and the developments in hair rejuvenation', *Int J Cosmet Sci*, **24** (2002), 1, 17–23

3. Bassett, I., Pannowitz, D. and Barnetson, R., 'A comparative study of tea-tree oil versus benzoylperoxide in the treatment of acne', *Med J Aust*, **153** (1990), 8, 455–8

4. Layton, A., 'Treatment of hyperandrogenism in PCOS', chapter in *Current Management of PCOS*, eds Balen, A. *et al.*, RCOG Press, 2010

5. Sinclair, R. *et al.*, 'Treatment of female pattern hair loss with oral antiandrogens', *Br J Dermatol*, **152** (2005), 3, 466–73

Chapter 9: Stress and PCOS

1. Selye, H., *The Stress of Life*, New York, McGraw Hill, 1978
2. Benson, S. *et al.*, 'Disturbed stress responses in women with PCOS', *Psychoneuroendocrinology*, **34** (2009), 5, 727–35
3. Gallinelli, I. *et al.*, 'Autonomic and neuroendocrine responses to stress in patients with functional hypothalamic secondary amenorrhea', *Fertil Steril*, **73** (2000), 4, 812–16
4. Epel, E.S. *et al.*, 'Stress and body shape: Stress-induced cortisol secretion is consistently greater among women with central fat', *Psychosomatic Medicine*, **62** (2000), 623–32
5. Epel, E.S. *et al.*, 'Stress may add bite to appetite in women: a laboratory study of stress-induced cortisol and eating behaviour', *Psychoneuroendocrinology*, **26** (2001), 1, 37–49
6. Hawley, G. *et al.*, 'Sustainability of health and lifestyle improvements following a non-dieting randomised trial in overweight women', *Prev Med*, **47** (2008), 6, 593–9
7. Segal, Z.V. *et al.*, 'Antidepressant monotherapy vs sequential pharmacotherapy and mindfulness-based cognitive therapy or placebo for relapse prophylaxis in recurrent depression', *Arch Gen Psychiatry*, **67** (2010), 12, 1256–64
8. Copinschi, G, 'Metabolic and endocrine effects of sleep deprivation', *Essent Psychopharmacol*, **6** (2005), 6, 341–7
9. Deckro, G.R. *et al.*, 'The evaluation of a mind/body intervention to reduce psychological distress and perceived stress in college students', *J Am Coll Health*, **50** (2002), 6, 281–7
10. Grewen, K.M. *et al.*, 'Effects of partner support on resting oxytocin, cortisol, norepinephrine, and blood pressure before and after warm partner contact', *Psychosomatic Medicine*, **67** (2005), 531–8
11. Deeks, A.A. *et al.*, 'Is having PCOS a predictor of poor psychological function including anxiety and depression?' *Hum Reprod*, **26** (2011), 6, 1399–407
12. Rofey, D.L. *et al.*, 'Cognitive behavioural therapy for physical and emotional disturbances in adolescents with PCOS: a pilot study', *J Pediatr Psychol*, **34** (2009), 2, 156–63

Chapter 10: Environmental Hormone Disruptors

1. Crisp, T.M. *et al.*, 'Environmental endocrine disruption: An effects assessment and analysis', *Environ Health Perspect*, **106** (Supp 1) (1998), 11–56
2. Diamanti-Kandarakis, E. *et al.*, 'Endocrine-Disrupting Chemicals: An Endocrine Society Scientific Statement', *Endocrine Reviews*, **30** (2009), 4, 293–342
3. Kandaraki, E. *et al.*, 'Endocrine disruptors and PCOS: elevated serum levels of bisphenol A in women with PCOS', *J Clin Endocrinol Metab*, **96** (2011), 3, E480–84
4. Sug, O. *et al.*, 'Exposure to bisphenol A is associated with recurrent miscarriage', *Hum Reprod*, **20** (2005), 8, 2325–9
5. Kandaraki, E. *et al.*, 'Endocrine disruptors and PCOS: elevated serum levels of bisphenol A in women with PCOS', *J Clin Endocrinol Metab*, **96** (2011), 3, E480–84
6. Fernandez, M. *et al.*, 'Neonatal exposure to Bisphenol A and reproductive and endocrine alterations resembling the polycystic ovarian syndrome in adult rats', *Environmental Health Perspectives*, **118** (2010), 9, 1217–22
7. Hoyer, P.B., 'Damage to ovarian development and function', *Cell Tissue Res*, **322** (2005), 1, 99–106
8. Pocar, P. *et al.*, 'The impact of endocrine disruptors on oocyte competence', *Reproduction*, **124** (2003), 3, 313–25
9. Rignell-Hydbom, A., 'Exposure to p, p'-DDE: a risk factor for type 2 diabetes', *PLoS One*, **4** (2009), 10, e7503
10. Lee, D.H. *et al.*, 'Low dose organochlorine pesticides and polychlorinated biphenyls predict obesity, dyslipidemia and insulin resistance among people free of diabetes', *PLoS One*, **6** (2011), 1, e15977
11. Bretveld, R.W. *et al.*, 'Pesticide exposure: the hormonal function of the female reproductive system disrupted?' *Reprod Biol Endocrinol*, **4** (31 May 2006), 30

Chapter 11: Your Fertility

1. Hudecova, M. *et al.*, 'Long-term follow-up of patients with polycystic ovary syndrome: reproductive outcome and ovarian reserve', *Human Reproduction*, **24** (2009), 5, 1176–83
2. Tehrani, F.R. *et al.*, 'Is PCOS an exception for reproductive ageing?' *Hum Reprod*, **25** (2010), 7, 1775–81
3. Chavarro, J.E. *et al.*, 'Diet and lifestyle in the prevention of ovulatory disorder infertility', *Obstet Gynecol*, **110** (2007), 5, 1050–58

4. Tolstrup, J.S. *et al.*, 'Alcohol use as predictor for infertility in a representative population of Danish women', *Act Obstet Gynecol Scand*, **82** (2003), 744–9

5. Guo, H. *et al.*, 'Effects of cigarette, alcohol consumption and sauna on sperm morphology', *Zhonghu Nan Ke Xue*, **12** (2006), 3, 215–17, 221

6. Lintsen, B., presented at the European Society of Human Reproduction and Embryology's annual conference, 2008

7. Weng, X. *et al.*, 'Maternal caffeine consumption during pregnancy and the risk of miscarriage: a prospective cohort study', *Am J Obstet Gynecol*, **198** (2008), 3, 279, e1–8

8. Nawrt, P. *et al.* 'Effects of caffeine on human health', *Food Addit Contam*, **20** (Jan 2003), 1, 1–30

9. Chavarro, J.E. *et al.*, 'Dietary fatty acid intakes and the risk of ovulatory infertility', *Am J Clin Nutr*, **85** (2007), 1, 231–7

10. Chavarro, J.E. *et al.*, 'Protein intake and ovulatory infertility', *Am J Obstet Gynecol*, **198** (2008), 2, 210, e1–7

11. ASH, 'Smoking and Reproduction', Research studies fact sheet, 2000

12. BMA report, 2004

13. Guo, H. *et al.*, 'Effects of cigarette, alcohol consumption and sauna on sperm morphology', *Zhonghua Nan Ke Xue*, **12** (2006), 3, 215–17, 221

14. Klonoff-Cohen, H. *et al.*, 'Effects of female and male smoking on success rates of IVF and gamete intra-fallopian transfer', *Human Reprod*, **16** (2001), 7, 1382–90

15. Sheynkin, Y. *et al.*, 'Increase in scrotal temperature in laptop computer users', *Hum Reprod*, **20** (2005), 2, 452–5

16. Hassan, M. *et al.*, 'Negative lifestyle is associated with a significant reduction in fecundity', *Fertil Steril*, **81** (2004), 384–92

17. Homan, G.F. *et al.*, 'The impact of lifestyle factors on reproductive performance in the general population and those undergoing fertility treatment: a review', *Hum Reprod Update*, **13** (2007), 3, 209–33

18. Chavarro, J.E. *et al.*, 'Use of multivitamins, intake of B vitamins and risk of ovulatory infertility', *Fertil Steril*, **89** (2008), 3, 668–76

19. Wong, W.Y., 'Effects of folic acid and zinc sulfate on male factor subfertility: a double-blind, randomized, placebo-controlled trial', *Fertil Steril*, **77** (2002), 3, 491–8

20. Safarinejad, M.R. and Safarinejad, S., 'Efficacy of selenium and/or N-acetyl-cysteine for improving semen parameters in infertile men: a double-blind, placebo controlled, randomized study', *J Urol*, **181** (2009), 2, 741–51

21. Greco, E. *et al.*, 'ICSI in cases of sperm DNA damage: beneficial effect of oral antioxidant treatment', *Hum Reprod*, **20** (2005), 9, 2590–94

22. Tarin, J. *et al.*, 'Effects of maternal ageing and dietary antioxidant supplementation on ovulation, fertilisation and embryo development in vitro in the mouse', *Reproduction, Nutrition, Development*, **38** (1998), 5, 499–508

23. Hayes, C.E. *et al.*, 'The immunological functions of the vitamin D endocrine system', *Cell Mol Biol*, **49** (2003), 2, 277–300

24. Panda, D.K. *et al.*, 'Targeted ablation of the 25-hydroxyvitamin D 1alpha - hydroxylase enzyme: evidence for skeletal, reproductive, and immune dysfunction', *Proc Natl Acad Sci USA*, **19** (2001), 98, 13, 7498–503

25. Blomberg Jensen, M. *et al.*, 'Vitamin D is positively associated with sperm motility and increases intracellular calcium in human spermatozoa', *Hum Reprod*, **26** (2011), 6, 1307–17

26. Srivastava, S., 'Mechanism of action of l-arginine on the vitality of spermatozoa is primarily through increased biosynthesis of nitric oxide', *Biol Reprod*, **74** (2006), 954–8

27. Gurbuz, B. *et al.*, 'Relationship between semen quality and seminal plasma total carnitine in infertile men', *J Obstet Gynae*, **23** (2003), 6, 653–6

28. Igarashi, M., 'Augmentative effect of ascorbic acid upon induction of human ovulation in clomiphene-ineffective anovulatory women', *Int J Fertil*, **22** (1977), 3, 168–73

29. Crha, I. *et al.*, 'Ascorbic acid and infertility treatment', *Cent Eur J Public Health*, **11** (2003), 2, 63–7

30. Akmal, M. *et al.*, 'Improvement in human semen quality after oral supplementation of vitamin C', *J Med Food*, **9** (2006), 3, 440–42

31. Showell, M.G. *et al.*, 'Antioxidants for male subfertility', *Cochrane Database Syst Rev* (2011), CD007411

32. Rossi, E. *et al.*, 'Fish oil derivatives as a prophylaxis of recurrent miscarriage associated with antiphospholipid antibodies (APL): a pilot study', *Lupus*, **2** (1993), 5, 319–23

33. Thies, F. *et al.*, 'Dietary supplementation with eicosapentaenoic acid, but not with other long-chain n-3 or n-6 polyunsaturated fatty acids, decreases natural killer cell activity in healthy subjects aged >55 y', *Am J Clin Nutr*, **73** (2001), 3, 539–48

34. Makhseed, M. *et al.*, 'Th1 and Th2 cytokine profiles in recurrent aborters with successful pregnancy and with subsequent abortions', *Hum Reprod*, **16** (2001), 2219–26

35. Ng, S.C. *et al.*, 'Expression of intracellular Th1 normal pregnancy', *Am J Reprod Immunol*, **48** (2002), 77–86
36. James, M.J. *et al.*, 'Dietary polyunsaturated fatty acids and inflammatory mediator production', *Am J Clin Nutr*, **71** (2000), 343S–8S
37. Aksoy, Y. *et al.*, 'Sperm fatty acid composition in subfertile men', *Prostaglandins Leukot Essent Fatty Acids*, **75** (2006), 2, 75–9
38. Safarinejad, M.R., 'Effect of omega-3 polyunsaturated fatty acid supplementation on semen profile and enzymatic anti-oxidant capacity of seminal plasma in infertile men with idiopathic oligoasthenoteratospermia: a double-blind, placebo-controlled, randomised study', *Andrologia*, **43** (2011), 1, 38–47
39. Kiddy, D.S. *et al.*, 'Improvement in endocrine and ovarian function during dietary treatment of obese women with polycystic ovary syndrome', *Clin Endocrinol*, **36** (1992), 105–11
40. Clark, A.M. *et al.*, 'Weight loss results in significant improvement in pregnancy and ovulation rates in anovulatory obese women', *Hum Reprod*, **10** (1995), 10, 2705–12
41. Clark, A.M. *et al.*, 'Weight loss in obese infertile women results in improvement in reproductive outcome for all forms of fertility treatment', *Human Reproduction*, **13** (1998), 6, 1502–5
42. Sallmen, M. *et al.*, 'Reduced fertility among overweight and obese men', *Epidemiology*, **17** (2006), 5, 520–23; and Kort, H. *et al.*, 'Impact of body mass index values on sperm quantity and quality', *J Androl*, **27** (2006), 3, 450–52
43. Stener-Victorin, E. *et al.*, 'Effects of electro-acupuncture on anovulation in women with PCOS', *Acta Obstet Gynecol Scand*, **79** (2000), 180–88
44. West, L. *et al.*, 'Acupuncture on the day of embryo transfer significantly improves reproductive outcome in infertile women: a prospective, randomized trial', *Fertil Steril*, **85** (2006), 5, 1341–6
45. Diet, S. *et al.*, 'Effect of acupuncture on the outcome of in vitro fertilization and intracytoplasmic sperm injection: a randomized, prospective, controlled clinical study', *Fertil Steril*, **85** (2006), 5, 1347–51
46. Gerhard, I. *et al.*, 'Individualised homeopathic therapy for male infertility', *Homeopathy*, **91** (Jul 2002), 3, 133–44
47. Bergman, J. *et al.*, 'The efficacy of the complex mediation phyto-hypophyson L in female, hormone-related sterility. A randomised placebo controlled clinical double blind study', *Forsch Komplementarmed Klass Naturheilkd*, **7** (2000), 4, 190–99
48. 'Has reflexology an effect on fertility?' Leila Eriksen, Chairman of the Forenede Danske Zneterapeuter (Danish Reflexology Association) Research Committee, 1994

49. 'Infertility and pregnancy loss – hypnotic interventions for reproductive challenges', in Hornyak L.M. *et al.* (eds), *The use of Hypnosis in women's health care*, The American Psychological Association, Washington DC, 2000

50. Gravitz, M.A., 'Hypnosis in the treatment of functional infertility', *Am J Clin Hypn*, **38** (1995), 1, 22–6

51. Levitas, E. *et al.*, 'Impact of hypnosis during embryo transfer on the outcome of in vitro fertilisation-embryo transfer: a case-control study', *Fertil Steril*, **85** (2006), 5, 1404–8

52. Perry, N. *et al*, 'Aromatherapy in the management of psychiatric disorders: clinical and neuropharmacological perspectives', *CNS Drugs*, **20** (2006), 4, 257–80

53. Thessalonki, ESHRE/ASRM-sponsored PCOS Consensus Workshop Group, 'Consensus on infertility treatment related to PCOS', *Hum Reprod*, **23** (2008), 2, 462–7

54. Homburg, R., 'Clomiphene citrate—end of an era? A mini-review', *Hum Reprod*, **20** (2005), 2043–51

55. Gysler, M. *et al.*, 'A decade's experience with an individualized clomiphene treatment regimen including its effects on the postcoital test', *Fertil Steril*, **37** (1982), 161–7

56. Nasseri, S. *et al.*, 'Clomiphene citrate in the twenty-first century', *Hum Fertil* (Camb), **4** (2001), 3, 145–51

57. Althuis, M.D. *et al.*, 'Uterine cancer after use of clomiphene citrate to induce ovulation', *Am J Epidemiol*, **161** (2005), 7, 607–11

58. Imani, B. *et al.*, 'Predictors of patients remaining anovulatory during clomiphene citrate induction of ovulation in normogonadotropic oligomenorrheic infertility', *J Clin Endocrinol Metab*, **83** (1998), 2361–5

59. Kosmas, I.P. *et al.*, 'Human chorionic gonadotrophin administration vs. luteinising monitoring for intrauterine insemination timing, after administration of clomiphene citrate: a meta-analysis', *Fertil Steril*, **87** (2007), 607–12

60. Tang, T. *et al.*, 'Insulin sensitising drugs (metformin, rosiglitazone, pioglitazone, D-chiro-inositol) for women with polycystic ovary syndrome, oligo amenorrhoea and subfertility', *Cochrane Database Syst Rev* (Online) (2010) (epub), no. 1, CD003053

61. *Current Management of PCOS*, eds Balen, A. *et al.*, RCOG Press, 2010

62. Badawy, A. *et al.*, 'Extended letrozole therapy for ovulation induction in clomiphene-resistant women with PCOS: a novel approach', *Fertil Steril*, **92** (2009), 236–9

63. Rizk, A.Y. *et al.*, 'N-acetyl cysteine is a novel adjuvant to clomiphene citrate in clomiphene citrate resistance patients with PCOS', *Fertil Steril*, **83** (2005), 2, 367–70

64. Shahin, A.Y. *et al.*, 'Adding phytoestrogens to clomiphene induction in unexplained infertility patients – a randomised trial', *Reprod Biomed Online*, **16** (2008), 4, 580–88

65. Eijkemans, M.J. *et al.*, 'High singleton live birth rate following classical ovulation induction in normogonadotrophic anovulatory infertility (WHO 2)', *Hum Reprod*, **18** (2003), 2357–62

66. Christin-Maitre, S. *et al.*, 'Comparative randomized multicentric study comparing the step-up versus step-down protocol in polycystic ovary syndrome', *Hum Reprod*, **18** (2003), 1626–31

67. American College of Obstetricians and Gynaecologists (2002, reaffirmed 2008), 'Management of infertility caused by ovulatory dysfunction', ACOG Practice Bulletin No. 34, *Obstetrics and Gynaecology*, **99** (2002), 2, 347–58

68. Palomba, S. *et al.*, 'Laparoscopic ovarian diathermy vs. clomiphene citrate plus metformin as second line strategy for infertility anovulatory patients with PCOS: a randomised controlled trial', *Am J Obstet Gynecol*, **202** (2010), 6, 577

69. Homburg, R., 'The management of infertility associated with PCOS', *Reprod Biol Endocrinol*, **1** (2003), 109

70. Nasr, A., 'Effect of N-acetyl-cysteine after ovarian drilling in clomiphene citrate-resistant PCOS women: a pilot study', *Reprod Biomed Online*, **20** (2009), 3, 403–9

71. Thessalonki, ESHRE/ASRM-sponsored PCOS Consensus Workshop Group, 'Consensus on infertility treatment related to PCOS', *Hum Reprod*, **23** (2008), 2, 462–7

72. Tang, T. *et al.*, 'The use of metformin for women with PCOS undergoing IVF treatment', *Hum Reprod*, **21** (2006), 1416–25

73. Stadtmauer, L.A. *et al.*, 'Metformin treatment of patients with PCOS undergoing IVF improves outcomes and is associated with modulation of the insulin-like growth factors', *Fertil Steril*, **75** (2001), 3, 50–59

74. Regan, L. *et al.*, 'Influence of past reproductive performance on risk of spontaneous abortion', *BMJ*, **299** (1989), 541–5

75. Jakubowicz, D.J. *et al.*, 'Effects of metformin on early pregnancy loss in the polycystic ovary syndrome', *J Clin Endocrinol Metab*, **87** (2002), 524–9

76. Vanky, E. *et al.*, 'Metformin versus placebo from first trimester to delivery in PCOS: a randomised controlled multicentre study', *J Clin Endocrinol Metab*, **95** (2010), 12, E448–55

77. Comhaire, F., 'The role of food supplementation in the treatment of the infertile couple and for assisted reproduction', *Andrologia*, **42** (2010), 5, 331–40

Chapter 12: Pregnancy
1. Boomsma, C.M. *et al.*, 'A meta-analysis of pregnancy outcomes in women with PCOS', *Hum Reprod Update*, **12** (2006), 673–83
2. Veltman-Verhulst, S.M. *et al.*, 'Sex hormone-binding globulin concentrations before conception as a predictor for gestational diabetes in women with polycystic ovary syndrome', *Hum Reprod*, **25** (2010), 12, 3123–8
3. Glueck, C.J. *et al.*, 'Prevention of gestational diabetes by metformin plus diet in patients with PCOS', *Fertil Steril*, **89** (2008), 625–34
4. Vanky, E. *et al.*, 'Metformin versus placebo from first trimester to delivery in PCOS: A randomised controlled multicentre study', *J Clin Endocrinol Metab*, **95** (2010), 12, E448–55
5. Thessalonki, ESHRE/ASRM-sponsored PCOS Consensus Workshop Group, 'Consensus on infertility treatment related to PCOS', *Hum Reprod*, **23** (2008), 2, 462–7
6. Bo, S. *et al.*, 'Gestational hyperglycemia, zinc, selenium and antioxidant vitamins', *Nutrition*, **21** (2005), 186–91
7. Das, U.N., 'Pathophysiology of metabolic syndrome X and its links to the perinatal period', *Nutrition*, **21** (2005), 762–73
8. Boomsma, C.M. *et al.*, 'A meta-analysis of pregnancy outcomes in women with PCOS', *Hum Reprod Update*, **12** (2006), 673–83
9. Maruotti, G. *et al.*, 'Pre-eclampsia and high serum levels of homocysteine', *Minerva Ginecol*, **57** (2005), 165–70
10. de Jager, J. *et al.*, 'Long term treatment with metformin in patients with type 2 diabetes and risk of vitamin B12 deficiency: randomised placebo controlled trial', *BMJ*, **340** (2010), c.2181
11. Saldeen, P. and Saldeen. T., 'Women and omega 3 fatty acids', *Obstet Gynecol Surv*, **59** (2004), 10, 722–30
12. William, M.A. *et al.*, 'Omega-3 fatty acids in maternal erythrocytes and risk of pre-eclampsia', *Epidemiology*, **6** (1995), 232–7
13. Hofmeyr, G.J. *et al.*, 'Calcium supplementation during pregnancy for preventing hypertensive disorders and related problems', *Cochrane Database Syst Rev*, **19** (2006), 3, CD001059
14. Casanueva, E. *et al.*, 'Vitamin C supplementation to prevent premature rupture of the chorioamniotic membranes: a randomised trial', *Am J Clin Nutr*, **81** (2005), 859–63

15. Olsen, S.F. and Secher, N.J., 'Low consumption of seafood in early pregnancy as a risk factor for preterm delivery: prospective cohort study', *BMJ*, **324** (2002), 447; and Allen, K.G. and Harris, M.A., 'The role of n-3 fatty acids in gestation and parturition', *Exp Biol Med* (Maywood), **226** (2001), 498–506

16. Morley, R. *et al.*, 'Maternal 25-hydroxyvitamin D and parathyroid hormone concentrations and offspring birth size', *J Clin Endocrinol Metab*, **91** (2006), 906–12

17. Scheplvagina, L.A., 'Impact of the mother's zinc deficiency on the woman's and newborn's health status', *J Trace Elem Med Biol*, **19** (2005), 29035

18. Nishijima, K. *et al.*, 'Probiotics affects vaginal flora in pregnant women, suggesting the possibility of preventing preterm labour', *J Clin Gastroenterol*, **39** (2005), 447–8

19. Nicoletto, S.F. and Rinaldi, A., 'In the womb's shadow. The theory of prenatal programming as the foetal origin of various adult diseases is increasingly supported by a wealth of evidence', *EMBO Rep*, **12** (2011), 1, 30–34

20. Meyer, K. *et al.*, 'Foetal programming of cardiac function and disease', *Reprod Sci*, **14** (2007), 3, 209–16

21. Kanaka-Gantenbein, C., 'Fetal origins of adult diabetes', *Ann NY Acad Sci*, **1205** (2010), 99–105

22. Sontrop, J. and Campbell, M.K., 'Omega 3 polyunsaturated fatty acids and depression: a review of the evidence and a methodological critique', *Prev Med*, **42** (2006), 4–130

23. Freeman, M.P. *et al.*, 'Randomised dose-ranging pilot trial of omega-3 fatty acids for postpartum depression', *Acta Psychiatr Scand*, **113** (2006), 31–5

24. Genuis, S.J. and Schwalfenberg, G.K., 'Time for an oil check: the role of essential Omega 3 fatty acids in maternal and pediatric health', *J Perinatol*, **26** (2006), 359–65

25. Helland, I.B. *et al.*, 'Maternal supplementation with very long chain n-3 fatty acids during pregnancy and lactation augments children's IQ at 4 years of age', *Pediatrics*, **111** (2003), e39–44

26. Dunstan, J.A. and Prescott, S.L., 'Does fish oil supplementation in pregnancy reduce the risk of allergic disease in infants?' *Curr Opin Allergy Clin Immunol*, **5** (2005), 215–21

Chapter 13: Nutritional Tests That Are Useful in Treating PCOS

1. Saldeen, P. and Saldeen, T., 'Women and omega 3 fatty acids', *Obstet Gynecol Surv*, **59** (2004), 10, 722–30

2. de Jager, J. *et al.*, 'Long term treatment with metformin in patients with type 2 diabetes and risk of vitamin B12 deficiency: randomised placebo controlled trial', *BMJ*, **340** (2010), c.2181

3. Maruotti, G. *et al.*, 'Pre-eclampsia and high serum levels of homocysteine', *Minerva Ginecol*, **57** (2005), 165–70

4. Setola, E. *et al.*, 'Insulin resistance and endothelial function are improved after folate and vitamin B12 therapy in patients with metabolic syndrome: relationship between homocysteine levels and hyperinsulinemia', *Eur J Endocrinol*, **15** (2004), 4, 483–9

Chapter 14: Safeguarding Your Future Health

1. Samy, N. *et al.*, 'Clinical significance of inflammatory markers in PCOS: their relationship to insulin resistance and body mass index', *Dis Markers*, **26** (2009), 163–70

2. Knowler, W.C. *et al.*, 'Ten year follow up of diabetes incidence and weight loss in the Diabetes Prevention Program Outcome Study', *Lancet*, **374** (2009), 1677–86

3. Wien, M. *et al.*, 'Almond consumption and cardiovascular risk factors in adults with prediabetes', *J Am Coll Nutr*, **29** (2010), 3, 189–97

4. Welsh, J.A. *et al.*, 'Caloric sweetener consumptions and dyslipidemia among US adults', *JAMA*, **303** (2010), 15, 1490–97

5. Setola, E. *et al.*, 'Insulin resistance and endothelial function are improved after folate and vitamin B12 therapy in patients with metabolic syndrome: relationship between homocysteine levels and hyperinsulinemia', *Eur J Endocrinol*, **15** (2004), 4, 483–9

6. de Jager, J. *et al.*, 'Long term treatment with metformin in patients with type 2 diabetes and risk of vitamin B12 deficiency: randomised placebo controlled trial', *BMJ*, **340** (2010), c.2181

7. Randeva, H.S. *et al.*, 'Exercise decreases plasma total homocysteine in overweight young women with polycystic ovary syndrome', *J Clin Endocrin Metab*, **87** (2002), 10, 4496–501

8. Giovannucci, E., 'The Role of Insulin Resistance and Hyperinsulinemia in Cancer', *Curr Med Chem*, **5** (2005), 1, 53–60

9. Fearnley, E.J. *et al.*, 'Polycystic ovary syndrome increases the risk of endometrial cancer in women aged less than 50 years: an Australian case-control study', *Cancer Causes Control*, **21** (2010), 12, 2303–8

10. Kabat, G.C. *et al.*, 'Repeated measures of serum glucose and insulin in relation to postmenopausal breast cancer', *Int J Cancer*, **125** (2009), 11, 2704–10

11. Eliassen, A.H. *et al.*, 'Adult weight change and risk of postmenopausal breast cancer', *JAMA*, **296** (2006), 193–201

12. Huang, Z. *et al.*, 'Waist circumference, waist hip ratio and risk of breast cancer in the Nurses' Health Study', *Am J Epidemol*, **150** (1999), 12, 1316–24

13. Lambrinoudaki, I., 'Cardiovascular risk in postmenopausal women with the PCOS', *Maturitas*, **68** (2011), 1, 13–16

14. Purrunen, J. *et al.*, 'Unfavorable hormonal, metabolic and inflammatory alternations persist after menopause in women with PCOS', *J Clin Endocrinol Metab*, **96** (2011), 6, 1827–34

15. Kassanos, D. *et al.*, 'Augmentation of cortical bone mineral density in women with PCOS: a peripheral quantitative computed tomography study', *Hum Reprod*, **25** (2010), 8, 2107–14

16. Schmidt, J. *et al.*, 'Reproductive hormone levels and anthropometry in postmenopausal women with polycystic ovary syndrome (PCOS): a 21-year follow-up study of women diagnosed with PCOS around 50 years ago and their age-matched controls', *J Clin Endocrinol Metab*, **96** (2011), 7, 2178–85

INDEX

acanthosis nigricans 10, 123, 127–8
acne 9, 10, 11, 15, 18, 19, 32–3, 49,
    51, 54, 55–6, 85, 123–4, 131,
    209
  medical treatment of 125–7
  natural treatment of 124–5
acrochordons 10, 123, 127
acupuncture 83, 170
adrenal glands 19–20, 27, 30, 41, 51,
    58, 59, 62, 99, 131, 160
  and diet supplements 71, 73
adrenaline 19, 100, 129, 130–1
aerobic (cardiovascular) exercise 107,
    108–11, 112
age 158–9, 164
agnus castus 80, 81, 82, 125
alcohol 41, 49, 56–7, 100, 160
aloe vera 124–5
alpha-lipoic acid 70, 74–5
amino acids 70, 76–7, 79, 82, 122,
    164, 176, 185–6, 196
anaerobic exercise 108, 111–12
androgenic alopecia see hair thinning
androgens 20, 26, 51, 93, 116, 123,
    131, 204, 210
anti-androgens 32–3, 128
androstenedione 20, 27
anti-mullerian hormone (AMH) 26,
    29
antibiotics 126–7
antioxidants 57, 74, 76, 163, 164,
    165, 184–5, 213
anxiety see mood swings; stress
appetite 74, 77, 79, 89–90, 91, 92,
    93, 95–6, 97, 99, 102
  food cravings 10, 16, 46, 47, 48, 70,
    73, 77, 97, 131, 142
  see also weight management
arginine 77, 164–5
aromatherapy 83, 100, 134, 171
aromatose inhibitors 176
autoimmune thyroid disease 89

bacteria, beneficial 33, 64, 72, 78, 79,
    125, 126–7
  see also probiotics
bariatric surgery 103
benzoyl peroxide 126
beta-carotene 213
binge eating 10, 90, 131, 141
biotin 70, 71–2, 120, 213
births, premature 186–8
bisphenol A (BPA) 149, 153
black cohosh 80–1, 82, 176
blood pressure 22, 49, 55, 196
  and pregnancy 184, 185–6
blood sugar levels 3, 14, 16, 41, 42,
    53, 56, 58, 83, 93, 95, 129, 199,
    200–1
  and diet supplement 70–1, 72, 73,
    74, 75, 77, 78, 79, 120
  dietary tips for balancing 44, 47–8,
    92, 98, 99–100, 120
  and exercise 107, 108
  and fertility 160, 161
  and stress 132–3
blood tests 26–8, 29–30, 36, 60, 64,
    73, 89, 164, 186, 187, 192–7,
    209
BMI (Body Mass Index) 86–7, 169,
    200
bone health 105, 204–5
branched-chain amino acids (BCAAs)
    79
breast cancer 203
breast tenderness 33, 69, 169
breathing techniques 136

C Reactive Protein (CRP) 61
Caesarean sections 184
caffeine 3, 41, 58–60, 99, 160–1
calcium 52–3, 67, 68, 72, 186,
    213
cancer 22, 53–4, 55, 59, 62, 174,
    193, 203–4

carbohydrates 3, 42, 43, 44, 45, 46,
71–2, 74, 93–4, 95, 99–100,
131, 185
  unrefined 41, 42–3, 54, 58, 132,
  160
carnitine 77, 164–5
cervical mucus 21, 167–8, 175, 179
chamomile tea 100
chemicals in the environment 147–50
  reducing your exposure to 150–4
cholesterol 27, 35, 36, 71, 91, 93,
95, 201
chromium 3, 46, 70–1, 133, 188, 214
clomiphene citrate (Clomid) 76, 105,
158, 165, 173, 174–6, 178
co-enzyme Q10 70, 74
coconut oil 92
cod-liver oil 78, 187
coffee 3, 59, 160–1
  see also caffeine
cognitive behavioural therapy (CBT)
143
coil, Mirena 82
comfort/emotional eating 97, 131,
141–2, 143
congenital adrenal hyperplasia 27
contraceptive Pill 3, 21–2, 28, 32–3,
34–5, 36, 69, 82, 92, 125
cortisol 19, 30, 58, 62, 95, 97, 99,
129, 130–1, 135, 195–6
counselling 144–5
cranial osteopathy 171–2
crash diets 87
cravings, food 10, 16, 46, 47, 48, 70,
73, 77, 97, 131, 142
cultural differences, PCOS and 21
Cushing's syndrome 30, 195–6, 210

D-chiro-inositol 72
dairy products 41, 50–5, 61, 160,
180
decaffeinated coffee 59
dehydroepiandrosterone sulphate
(DHEAS) 20, 27, 195
depression 1, 10, 138, 143
  see also stress
diabetes 22, 27, 34, 44, 49, 51, 55,
59, 63, 72, 73, 76, 88, 149, 176,
184, 189, 200–1
  gestational 183–4, 200

Dianette 32–3, 125
diaries, food 96
diet 3, 11, 34, 213–16
  calcium 52–3
  carbohydrates 3, 41, 42–4, 45, 46,
  54, 58, 71–2, 74, 93–4, 95,
  99–100, 131, 132, 160, 185
  dairy products 41, 50–5, 61, 160,
  180
  environmental chemicals 151–2
  fibre 44, 45, 72, 92
  foods to help with weight loss
  90–4
  Omega 3 fats and oily fish 41,
  49–50, 54–5, 60, 61, 62, 68, 76,
  160, 165–6, 187, 194–5, 214
  proteins 3, 41, 42, 45, 76, 92–3,
  112, 120, 161, 180
  resistant starch 93–4
  saturated fats 41, 61–2, 160, 185
  seven-steps to beat PCOS 39–65,
  160
  trans fats 41, 62–3, 160
  see also drinks; supplements; weight
  management
dihydrotestosterone (DHT) 51
dioxins 50, 78
discolouration, skin 10, 123, 127–8
diuretics 33, 57, 58, 128
drugs, prescribed see medications

eating habits 47–8, 95–8, 99, 137–8,
141–3, 144–5
  see also cravings; diet; weight
  management
echinacea 125
eggs, human 12–13, 14, 15, 21, 26,
29, 72, 105, 149, 174, 178–80,
181
electrolysis 118
emotional issues 138–41, 143–4
  and eating behaviours 141–3
endometrial cancer 22
endometrial hyperplasia 19
endorphins 105, 136
energy levels see tiredness
environmental chemicals 147–50
  reducing your exposure to 150–4
epilation 117
erythromycin 126

essential fatty acids 49, 63, 75, 165, 214
see also Omega 3 fats and oily fish
evening primrose oil 60, 166, 194
exercise 11, 34, 53, 75, 100, 105–8, 112–13, 203
  aerobic exercise with interval training 108–11, 112
  anaerobic exercise with resistance training 108, 111–12
  to help stress 135–6

fallopian tubes 12, 172–3
fasting glucose 26, 28
fats 71, 95
  around middle of body 57, 61, 62, 63, 79, 92, 106, 131, 196, 203–4
  burning 58, 76, 77, 87, 91, 107, 109–10, 111, 112–13
  polyunsaturated 60–1
  saturated 41, 61–2, 160, 185
  trans fats 62–3, 160, 161
  see also Omega 3 fats and oily fish
ferritin 120–1
fertility *see* infertility
fibre 44, 45, 72, 92
fight or flight response 130–1
finger-prick tests
  for homocysteine levels 186, 196–7, 203
  Omega 3/6 ration test 60, 194–5
  for vitamin D 64, 73, 89, 164, 187, 192–4
fish, oily *see* Omega 3 fats and oily fish
flaxseed (linseeds) 49, 55, 76, 121, 160, 166, 188
folic acid 3, 163, 186, 188, 197, 202, 214
follicle-stimulating hormone (FSH) 14, 15, 26, 28, 30, 174, 177, 178, 180, 181
follicles 9, 12, 14, 15, 20, 29, 51, 72, 85, 149, 159, 174, 175, 176, 180
free androgen index (FAI) 26
'free' foods 45
fructooligosaccharides (FOS) 78
fruit 44, 67–8, 91–2, 152, 185

gastric bands 103
genes 11–12, 88–9
gestational diabetes 183–4, 200
ghrelin 89–90, 91, 99
ginseng, Siberian 70, 80, 82, 133, 196
glucagon 77
glucose 16–17, 26, 27, 28, 34, 42, 45, 49, 50, 51, 70–1, 72, 73, 74, 75–6, 91, 93, 107, 176, 184
  see also blood sugar levels
glucose tolerance factor (GTF) 70–1
glutamine 77
glycaemic index (GI) 43, 53, 54, 78, 91, 92, 93, 98
goal setting 140
grains 44, 70, 72, 92
green tea 58, 70, 80, 82, 91

hair
  direct treatments of excess 116–19
  excess body and facial 2, 3, 4, 9, 10, 15, 18, 19, 21, 32–3, 49, 51, 56, 85, 115–19, 128, 209, 210
  loss of 10, 15, 71, 119–23, 128, 131
heart 49, 105
  disease/strokes 22, 55, 57, 59, 62, 63, 186, 189, 201–2, 204
herbs 2, 64, 69, 158
  agnus castus 3, 81, 82, 125
  to aid sleep 101
  black cohosh 3, 80–1, 82, 176
  combination supplements 80
  echinacea 125
  to help with hair loss 121
  to help with skin problems 125
  milk thistle 3, 80, 81
  saw palmetto 80, 81
  Siberian ginseng 70, 80, 82, 133
  tips for choosing 80
  warnings about 69, 82
herpes 77
high blood pressure 184–5, 196, 201
hirsutism 11, 34, 51, 115–16, 209, 210
  direct treatments for 116–19
  see also hair
homeopathy 83, 170
homocysteine 185–6, 196–7, 201–3

hormones 1, 2, 4, 9, 12–13, 41, 42, 57, 65, 68, 83, 101, 170, 171
  adrenaline 19, 100, 129, 130–1
  androgens 20, 26, 51, 93, 116, 119–20, 123, 131, 204
  and appetite 89–90, 91, 95, 99
  and the contraceptive Pill 28, 32–3, 34–5, 36, 69, 82, 92, 125
  cortisol 19, 30, 58, 62, 95, 97, 99, 129, 130–1, 135, 195–6
  and diet supplements 71, 72, 73, 74, 75, 77
  environmental disruption of 147–8
  FSH 14, 15, 26, 28, 30, 174, 177, 178, 180, 181
  and herbs 69, 80, 81, 82
  luteinizing hormones (LH) 3, 11, 14, 15, 17, 19, 20, 26, 28, 30, 35, 80, 167–8, 174, 178, 181
  male (general) 11, 17, 19, 20, 21, 25, 26, 27, 33, 35, 41, 49, 51, 53, 54, 72, 81, 82, 106, 116, 119–20, 123, 125, 130, 160, 175, 209, 210–11 (*see also* androgens; testosterone)
  oestrogen 14, 17, 18–19, 57, 58, 62, 131, 174–5, 203
  progesterone 14, 15, 27, 30, 32, 89, 176
  and SHBG 17, 20, 21, 26, 55, 93
  stress (general) 19–20, 48, 129–31, 132, 135–6, 137 (*see also* adrenaline; cortisol)
  testing levels of 26–8, 29–30
  testosterone 15, 17, 18, 19, 20, 21, 26, 28, 32, 34, 35, 50, 51, 54, 55, 75, 81, 85, 129, 131, 149, 177
  and your weight 18–19, 85–6
  see also insulin
horsetail 121
HyCoSy (hystero-contrast sonography) 172, 173
hydration 112
hypertension 184–5
  see also blood pressure
hypnotherapy 83, 141, 143–4, 171
hysterosalpingogram (HSG) 172

ICSI (intracytoplasmic sperm injection) 180–1

IGF-1 50–1, 54
immune system 62, 64, 75, 105, 124, 125, 164, 165, 166
infertility 1, 2, 9, 10, 11, 63, 131, 149
  and exercise 105–6
  lifestyle tips for boosting fertility 159–62
  medical treatments for 36, 76, 173–80 (*see also* clomiphene citrate; IVF)
  natural therapies 169–72, 182
  supplements to boost fertility 33, 162–6
  tests 172–3
  and weight 85, 169
  see also miscarriages; ovulation; pregnancy
inflammation 14, 35, 41, 61–2, 63, 64, 82, 90, 106, 124, 125, 126, 185, 189, 194, 196, 199–200
  and diet supplements 71, 72, 73, 74, 75, 76, 79, 164, 165
inositol 70, 72
insulin 11, 19, 39, 44, 45, 47, 53, 54, 55, 58, 62, 82, 83, 85, 96, 129, 199–200
  and diet supplements and herbs 64, 70–1, 72, 73, 74, 75, 76, 77, 82, 164, 165
  and exercise 105, 107
  and IGF-1 50–1
  resistance 13–14, 15–17, 18, 20, 21, 22, 33, 34–5, 36, 41, 42, 49, 51, 61, 63, 70–1, 72, 73, 77, 79, 91–2, 99, 105, 107, 127, 135, 149, 184, 197, 201–2, 203
  sensitisers 34–5, 36, 40, 51, 102, 158 (*see also* metformin)
  sensitivity 34–5, 51, 58, 63, 64, 72, 76, 77, 83, 91, 92, 93, 105, 112
iodine 214
IPL (intense pulsed light) 119
iron 67–8, 120, 121–2, 188, 214
isotretinoin, oral (Roaccutane) 127
IUI (intrauterine insemination) 178
IVF (in-vitro fertilization) 2, 29, 158–9, 161, 165, 166, 169, 170, 171, 178–9
IVM (in-vitro maturation) 29, 181

laparoscopy 173
laser hair removal 118–19
lauric acid 92
legumes 44, 72
leptin 74, 89, 90, 95, 97, 99
letrozole 176
libido 10
linseeds (flaxseeds) 49, 55, 76, 121, 160, 166, 188
lipid profile 27
liver 3, 16, 20, 34, 35, 36, 41, 55, 56–7, 74, 81, 92, 95
luteinizing hormone (LH) 3, 11, 14, 15, 17, 19, 20, 26, 28, 30, 35, 80, 167–8, 174, 178, 181
lysine 122

magnesium 49, 67, 70, 71, 73, 74, 78, 98, 101, 133, 188, 196, 214
maltodextrin 78
manganese 70, 74, 188, 214
meat 61, 68, 185
medications 2, 31–6, 39, 64, 71, 75, 76, 82, 92, 102, 105
  for fertility 76, 105, 158, 165, 173, 174–6, 178
  for skin problems 125–8
  slimming drugs 102
  to treat hair loss 122–3
  see also contraceptive Pill; IVF; metformin
meditation 134
menopause 30, 203, 204–5, 210
menstrual cycle 2, 3–4, 10–11, 12–13, 14–15, 22, 26, 28, 32–3, 34–5, 85, 168, 210, 211
  diet supplements and herbs 68–9, 72, 77, 81, 125
  see also ovulation
mercury 50, 78
metabolism 48, 71, 73, 74, 77, 86, 87, 92, 96, 113
metformin 34–5, 36, 39, 64, 71, 75, 102, 120, 158, 176, 180, 181, 184, 186, 196, 202
methionine 185–6, 196
milk 51, 53–5, 68, 180
milk thistle 3, 80, 81
mindfulness based cognitive therapy 135

minerals (general) 33, 53, 67–8, 70, 78, 122, 158
  see also supplements; individual minerals by name
minoxidil (Regaine) 122–3
Mirena coil 33, 82
miscarriages 10, 64, 76, 149, 161, 163, 166, 169, 176, 178, 181
mood swings 10, 48, 69
MOOM wax 117–18
MRI scans 30
multivitamins and minerals 3, 36, 53, 70, 71–2, 73, 124, 162, 186, 188, 193, 202
  see also supplements
muscle building 77, 87, 106, 107–8, 111, 113

N-acetyl cysteine 76, 176, 178
NLP (neurolinguistic programming) 144
nocturnal hypoglycaemia 99–100
Nutri Support 75
nutritional tests 191, 218
  adrenal stress tests 195–6
  homocysteine 186, 196–7, 203
  Omega 3/6 ration test 60, 194–5
  vitamin D 64, 73, 89, 164, 187, 192–4

obesity see weight management
oestrogen 14, 17, 18–19, 57, 58, 62, 131, 174–5, 178, 203, 204
OHSS (ovarian hyperstimulation syndrome) 175, 180, 181
Omega 3 fats and oily fish 41, 49–50, 54–5, 60, 61, 62, 68, 76, 158, 160, 165–6, 187, 194–5, 214
  supplements 70, 75, 121, 125, 158, 162, 165–6, 186, 187, 188, 189
Omega 6 fats 60–1, 75, 194–5, 214
organic food 54–5, 62, 152, 160
Orlistat 102
osteopathy 83, 171–2
osteoporosis 204
ovaries 11, 27, 34, 85, 159
  cancer 53–4
  and the contraceptive Pill 21–2
  development of PCOS 12–13
  drilling surgery 76, 177–8

ovaries (*cont.*)
  and environmental chemicals 149
  herbs and supplements 72, 81
  and IGF-1 51, 54
  medical infertility treatment 29,
    105, 174–5, 177, 179–80, 181
  and menstrual cycle 14–15, 26, 72
  testosterone production 17, 19, 20,
    129
  ultrasound scans 12, 22, 28–9,
    210–11
  and weight loss 169
ovulation 10, 11, 15, 20, 21–2, 26,
    28, 34, 36, 63, 72, 76, 77, 85,
    105, 161, 164, 174, 175–6, 178,
    209, 210
  ways to check you are ovulating
    167–9
  see also infertility
oxytocin 137

Panax ginseng 82
pancreas 13–14, 17, 42, 47, 70, 107
PCBs (polychlorinated biphenyls) 50,
    78
periods *see* menstrual cycle
pesticides/insecticides 151–2, 154
phytoestrogens 215
Pill, contraceptive 3, 21–2, 28, 32–3,
    34–5, 36, 69, 82, 92, 125
pituitary glands 14, 15, 17, 26, 30,
    81, 137
PMS (pre-menstrual syndrome) 60
polycystic ovary syndrome (PCOS)
    1–5, 9–11, 15–19, 207–8
  causes of 11–12
  cultural differences 21
  diagnosing 25–30, 209–11
  and environmental chemicals
    147–9
  and genes 88–9
  how it develops 12–13
  medical treatment of 31–6
  overview of symptoms 10–11
  seven-step diet 39–65, 160
  and surgery 36, 76, 177–8
  and thyroid function 89
  'vicious cycle' of 20–1
  see also acne; diet; exercise; hair;
    hormones; insulin resistance;

ovaries; stress; supplements;
    weight management
polyphenol catechins 59
polyunsaturated fats 60–1
postnatal depression 189
pre-eclampsia 185–6, 196
pregnancy 50, 64, 76, 77, 164, 175,
    189
  and gestational diabetes 183–4, 200
  high blood pressure and pre-
    eclampsia 185–6
  preterm delivery 186–8
  supplements 184–5, 186, 187–8,
    189
  see also infertility; miscarriages;
    sperm
premature births 186–8
probiotics 64, 70, 78, 79, 125, 127,
    188
progesterone 14, 15, 32, 89, 176
  17-OH 27, 30
prolactin 26, 30
prostaglandins 61, 73, 166
proteins
  pre-eclampsia 185
  SHBG 17, 20, 21, 26, 32, 41, 44,
    54, 55, 56, 85, 93, 184
  in your diet 3, 41, 42, 45, 76,
    92–3, 112, 120, 161, 180, 215

reflexology 83, 170–1
Regaine (minoxidil) 122–3
relaxation 134–5
resistant starch 93–4
resveratrol 57
retinoids, topical 127
Roaccutane 127
Rotterdam Criteria 210

saliva tests 30
saturated fats 41, 61–2, 160, 185
saw palmetto 80, 81
scales, weighing 87–8
scans, ultrasound 22, 28–9, 167,
    175, 179, 210–11
sebum production 123, 125, 127
selenium 163, 184–5, 188, 215
self-esteem 139–41, 143
semen *see* sperm
sex drive 10

SHBG (sex hormone-binding globulin) 17, 20, 21, 26, 32, 41, 44, 54, 55, 56, 85, 93, 184
Siberian ginseng 70, 80, 82, 133, 196
Sibutramine 102
silica 121
skin 120, 121
  acne 2, 3, 9, 10, 11, 15, 18, 19, 32–3, 49, 51, 54, 55–6, 85, 123–7, 131
  discolouration 10, 123, 127–8
  and environmental chemicals 150–1
  tags 10, 123, 127
sleep 16, 99–101, 135
slimming drugs 102
smoking 161
soya 44, 49
sperm 158, 160, 163, 164, 166, 167, 169, 170, 173, 178–9, 180–1
spironolactone 128
spotting during ovulation 169
starch, resistant 93–4
statins 35, 36
Stein-Leventhal syndrome 9
  see also polycystic ovary syndrome (PCOS)
stress 19–20, 30, 49, 73, 80, 82, 97–8, 106, 120, 129–30, 171
  adrenal stress tests 195–6
  and balancing blood sugar 132–3
  dealing with emotional issues 138–41, 143–5
  and eating habits 141–3, 144–5
  practical ways to deal with 133–8
  supplements to treat 133
sugar 3, 42, 46–7, 49, 70, 77, 95, 160
superfoods 215
supplements 2, 64, 68–9, 103, 158, 218
  alpha-lipoic acid 70, 74–5
  amino acids 70, 76–7, 79, 122, 164, 176, 178
  B vitamins 70, 71–2, 74, 78, 98, 120, 133, 163, 188, 201–2
  biotin 70, 71, 120
  calcium 186, 188
  chromium 3, 46, 70–1, 133, 188, 214

co-enzyme Q10 70, 74
evening primrose oil 60, 166, 194
folic acid 163, 186, 188
inositol 70
iron 122, 188
magnesium 70, 71, 73, 74, 98
manganese 70, 74, 188
multivitamins and minerals 3, 36, 53, 70, 73, 124, 162, 186, 188, 193, 202
Omega 3 fats and fish-oil 70, 75, 121, 125, 158, 162, 165–6, 186, 187, 188, 189, 194–5
probiotics 64, 70, 78, 79, 127, 188
resveratrol 57
selenium 163, 188
to support
  adrenal glands 71, 73
  fertility 162–6
  hair regrowth 120–1
  inflammation reduction 71, 72, 73, 74, 75, 76, 79, 164, 165
  menstrual cycles 68–9, 72, 77, 81, 125
  pregnancy 184–5, 186, 187–8
  to treat stress 133
  treatment of acne 124, 125
  weight loss 64, 71, 72, 74, 76, 77, 79
tips for choosing 69, 78
Tranquil Woman 133
vitamin C 70, 75–6, 78, 122, 162, 164, 165, 176, 187, 188
vitamin D 64–5, 70, 72–3, 78, 164, 187, 188, 193
vitamin E 78, 164, 188
zinc 70, 71, 73–4, 122, 124, 163, 187–8
see also herbs; individual vitamins and minerals by name
support groups 145, 217–18
surgery 31, 36–7, 76, 103, 177–8
sweeteners, artificial 47, 95, 160

Tabata 109–10
t'ai chi 106
tamoxifen 176
tea 58–9, 99, 122, 162
  see also green tea
tea tree oil 124

temperature and ovulation 168
testosterone 15, 17, 18, 19, 20, 21,
    26, 28, 32, 34, 35, 50, 51, 54,
    55, 75, 81, 85, 129, 131, 149,
    177
tests for PCOS 25–30, 209–11
tetracycline 126
'thrifty' genes 88–9
thyroid function 26, 30, 71, 74, 77,
    89, 120
tiredness 3, 16, 48, 58, 120
toxins 50, 78, 112, 163, 164, 165,
    185–6, 196
  chemicals in the environment 147–50
  reducing your exposure to 150–4
Tranquil Woman 133
trans fats 41, 62–3, 160, 161
tryptophan 100
TSH (thyroid-stimulating hormone)
    26, 30
tyrosine 77

ultrasound scans 22, 28–9, 167, 175,
    179, 210–11
unrefined carbohydrates 41, 42–3,
    54, 58, 132, 160, 185
urine tests 30

Vaniqa cream 118
vegetables and pulses 3, 41, 44, 55–6,
    57, 67–8, 152, 160, 161, 185
Verity – PCOS support group 145
visualization techniques 101, 135
vitamin A 73–4, 102, 127, 187, 188,
    215
vitamin B (family) 70, 71–2, 74, 78,
    98, 120, 133, 163, 188, 201–2
vitamin B1 215
vitamin B2 70, 71, 215
vitamin B3 70, 71, 215
vitamin B5 70, 71, 196, 216
vitamin B6 49, 70, 71, 74, 78, 186,
    197, 216
vitamin B12 36, 71, 120, 163, 186,
    196, 197, 202–3, 216
vitamin C 70, 75–6, 78, 122, 162,
    164, 165, 176, 187, 216
vitamin D 64–5, 70, 72–3, 78, 89,
    90, 102, 164, 187, 192–4, 216
  nutritional test for 192–3

vitamin D2 78
vitamin D3 78, 187
vitamin E 73–4, 78, 101, 102, 164,
    216
vitamins (general) 33, 36, 158

water 112, 142
water retention 33, 185
waxing 117–18
weight management 3, 11, 21, 28,
    44, 45–6, 49, 68, 73, 82, 85–7
  BMI 86–7, 169, 200
  comfort/emotional eating 97, 131,
    141–2
  crash diets 87
  and diet supplements 64, 71, 72,
    74, 76, 77, 79
  eating habits 47–8, 95–8, 99,
    141–3, 144–5
  fat around middle of body 61, 62,
    63, 79, 92, 106, 196, 203–4
  fat burning 58, 76, 77, 87, 91, 107,
    109–10, 111, 112–13
  food diaries 96–7, 143
  foods to help aid weight loss 90–4
  gastric bands 103
  and infertility 169–70
  PCOS and weight gain 9, 10,
    16–17, 18–19, 34, 42, 57, 85–6
  and relaxation techniques 135
  resistant starch 93–4
  scales and measuring 87–8
  and sleep 99
  slimming drugs 102
  see also diet; drinks; exercise; insulin
    resistance
wheat 70, 94
wombs 11, 174, 203
  fertility treatments 170, 172, 176,
    178–9, 194
  lining 14, 19, 21, 22, 32, 175, 176,
    178

Yasmin 33
yoga 106, 135

zinc 3, 33, 49, 58, 68, 70, 71, 73–4,
    122, 124, 160, 163, 184–5,
    187–8, 216